Pelvic Pain Game Changer

6 STEPS TO
A HEALTHIER YOU

PELVIC PAIN
GAME
CHANGER

CAROLYN MARTHANÓIR

NEW YORK

LONDON • NASHVILLE • MELBOURNE • VANCOUVER

Pelvic Pain Game Changer

6 Steps to a Healthier You

Published in New York, New York, by Morgan James Publishing in partnership with Difference Press. Morgan James is a trademark of Morgan James, LLC. www.MorganJamesPublishing.com

ISBN 9781631950612 paperback
ISBN 9781631950629 eBook
Library of Congress Control Number: 2020934155

Cover Design Concept:
Nakita Duncan

Cover Design by:
Megan Dillon
megan@creativeninjadesigns.com

Interior Design by:
Christopher Kirk
www.GFSstudio.com

Editor:
Cory Hott

Book Coaching:
The Author Incubator

Interior Graphic Art Designs by:
Cindi Duft
www.cindiduft.com

Author Photo:
Lori Diane Fowlkes

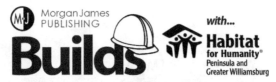

Morgan James is a proud partner of Habitat for Humanity Peninsula and Greater Williamsburg. Partners in building since 2006.

Get involved today! Visit
MorganJamesPublishing.com/giving-back

For all who suffer from an invisible or incurable disease seeking answers and relief. May you find comfort and joy and be free from pain.

Table of Contents

Chapter 1:

At the Game Table

"If there is no struggle, there is no progress."
– Frederick Douglass,
West Indian Emancipation Speech (1857)

Imagine for a moment that you are going to the grocery store to pick up a few things while your daughter is taking a lesson at the dance studio. You have your cart and you're going up and down each aisle, picking up an item here and there—a bag of potatoes, a jar of pickles—and all of sudden you feel a sharp, stabbing pain in your abdomen and a whoosh of warm ooze exiting your body, starting to run down your legs.

Panic sets in. "Oh my gosh," you think. "Not now."

Making your way to the back of the store to the restrooms, you keep your legs clenched together and waddle into the bathroom stall. You look in your purse.

"Thank you, Lord," you think as you pull a spare pad and wipes out of your bag. As you make your way down to the seat, it all gushes out—a blood clot the size of your fist along with some blood. You stand up and begin to clean yourself up with the wipes, but then start to feel light-headed. You need to get out of there.

You stick the pad to the inside of your pants—yes, you learned that you should always wear black—and then you wrap your panties in some paper towels and carefully place it inside your purse. Washing your hands, you look up at the mirror. You look pale, like a ghost. Yes, you feel like you're dying, or maybe you are already half-dead.

"Why can't doctors figure out what is wrong with me?" You wonder. "This can't be normal." You exit the bathroom and find your cart waiting for you. Thankfully, you never made it to the freezer or refrigerator sections, or all your frozen food would be melting. You leave the cart, as now you have lost your appetite. In fact, you feel a bit nauseous and are not in the mood to finish your shopping. There is a pizza place next to the dance studio, so you can pick up a pizza for the kids to eat.

While you are sitting in your car, waiting for your daughter's class to be over, you look at the calendar on your phone. It's the tenth, and your period doesn't normally start until the twentieth. What is going on?

Your daughter walks up to the car and gets in. She instantly sees that you aren't okay and asks, "What's wrong?" You tell her what you always tell her: that your stomach hurts and you just need to lie down for a little bit. You start the car and make your way home.

Once you are safely home, the kids are naturally happy to have pizza and you make your way upstairs to the bathroom. There, you open the medicine cabinet. Most homes have the little mirrored cabinet by the sink, but not you. Your medicine cabinet is two of the three shelves of what most people would use as a linen closet, showcasing your collection of the various medications that doctors prescribed to treat your symptoms. However, you just grab the ibuprofen and take four capsules, change your pants, and lie down on the bed with your heating pad. You can feel the pain radiating down your legs, almost in waves. You close your eyes and internally rock with the waves, go with the flow, and be with your pain. You ask your body, "What's wrong?" But it doesn't answer. Clearly, it's upset about something. You wonder, "What did we do to upset the applecart today?"

An hour later, you wake up to the sound of your husband coming into the room. "What's going on?" he asks, and you can tell by the sound of his voice that he is frustrated, probably due to the fact that he came home from work to find the kids, who are eleven and eight, eating pizza, camped out in front of the television while you are upstairs in bed, curled up in the fetal position with your heating pad.

The truth is, you can't answer the question, "What is going on?" because you don't know the answer. The doctors don't seem to know. All you know is what you feel and that is all you can share.

You tell him about the episode in the grocery store, and that you noticed that your cycle is off. But the thing is, you have been telling him similar stories ever since your daughter was born eight years ago. The episodes are just becoming more frequent and more painful. He's getting tired of it, and so are you.

"So, what are you going to do about it?" he asks.

"I'm going to call the doctor's office in the morning and see if I can get in." Maybe we will get some answers this time. You can only hope and pray because you have been down this road before. You have been to dozens of different doctors, had dozens of lab tests, and did dozens of pelvic exams that left you feeling violated and in pain, and they accomplished no results. You are just not sure how much longer you can meander down this path.

You are tired.

You are tired of the pain.

You are tired of the doctors' appointments and the poking and prodding.

You are tired of not getting any answers.

You are tired of the judgments, of being labeled as "lazy," "no fun," "energy-draining," "unreliable," "fat," "angry," or "depressed."

You are tired of strangers asking, "When is your baby due?" and you are not even pregnant.

If only these people could spend a day in your body and feel what you feel, and experience what you experience. Then they might understand. But this isn't their game to play - it's yours. We must play with the cards we are dealt, just like we can't change the structure or sequence of our DNA. However, we do have the ability to influence the expression of our genes. It's all in how you play the cards you are dealt.

That is why I wrote this book: to help women, who feel helpless with undiagnosed chronic pelvic pain and to share with them what I have learned to find the cause and the remedy to their pain.

Chapter 2:

How Did I Get Here?

"The cost of a thing is the amount of what I will call life, which is required to be exchanged for it, immediately or in the long run."
– Henry David Thoreau, *Walden, Economy (1854)*

I consider myself an average female American, with a relatively humble upbringing. I was born in the "great potato state" of Idaho, the first of four children born to parents of Swiss-German and Baltic ancestry. I was raised with familial traditions. My father's family came to America with a Catholic monk in the 1890s, and I graduated from the only Catholic high school in Idaho. It was pretty much a foregone conclusion that after graduating from high school, I would get married and have kids, but I had an incredible sense of wanderlust and had only been to seven of the fifty states—Idaho and its surrounding states. Getting married and having kids seemed boring. "Everybody does that," I thought. I knew there was a much bigger world out there and I wanted to travel and experience the places that I read about in books or saw on the big screen.

A few years after graduating high school, I was employed by an airline and my adventures began. I met and worked with so many amazing people and visited new and exciting places with different types of food, languages, music, and customs. At the same time, I felt my internal clock ticking. I wanted to have kids. I wanted to have a husband. My twenties were almost over, and I considered that it might be time to start a new journey.

After all, my boyfriend asked me to marry him. I lived in Maryland, worked at BWI Airport, and my boyfriend just graduated from the U.S. Navy's Officer Candidate School in Pensacola, Florida. At that point, we knew each other for about two years. We originally planned to wait a couple more years before considering the idea of marriage to see if we could survive the "long-distance" relationship. But it was my boyfriend, Guy, who said in one of our many marathon phone conversations, "We know we are going to be together; we are happier when we are together. Why are we waiting?"

I remember reflecting on that. Every time I visited Guy in Florida or Tennessee and then had to get on a plane to head back to Maryland, my heart felt tortured. I didn't want to leave because I loved being with him. The answer I gave Guy when he proposed was, "Yes." The date was set in-between his duty stations in Tennessee and Georgia. We got married on September 30, 2000, in the same Catholic church my parents got married in and where I was baptized. I left my career of seven years in the airline industry to become a transient military spouse.

One could say that because Guy wore his dress white Navy uniform at our wedding that I should have known what I was getting into. I was used to traveling—I liked to travel. I was used to having a long-distance relationship over the phone. I lived alone for ten years. I was independent, so I thought I could handle a military marriage. Honestly, the hardest thing was having to start over again every time we moved, and we moved four times in the first four years of our marriage. Every time you move, it means finding a new house, new job, new friends, new doctors, and learning the new "law of the land," as far as the rules with each new location and its military command.

After attending some counseling sessions, I learned that having difficulty with adapting to so many "life changes" at once is normal. Everyone experiences some anxiety about moving and getting their bearings in a new environment. I moved a lot with the airlines, but

I couldn't figure out why these moves were different. I then realized it was because I was mentally prepared for the other moves. The military was never forthcoming with information and I was a planner. Everything always seemed last minute and rushed when it came to military moves. Quite often, we didn't even know where we were going to be living until the day the moving van showed up. My counselor also highlighted some other "life-changing" events that occurred in those first four years that were even more significant.

September 11 changed my life forever because the military base we lived on went on high alert. My husband went out to sea immediately and I didn't know where he was going or when he would be back. We became a country at war. Living at the New London Submarine Base in Connecticut, we weren't that far from the destruction that occurred in New York City. In fact, we could see the smoke in the air for several days afterward. As a former airline employee, I also felt a personal connection to the events of that day.

Another significant event that happened that same year was my father's terminal cancer diagnosis and death. My father lived for eight months after his diagnosis of mucinous adenocarcinoma, and he died the Tuesday before Thanksgiving of that year. Since my husband was out to sea for much of the year, I was able to spend some time visiting and helping my parents. I think the hardest part for me was seeing my father—whom a little girl often envisions as being the biggest, strongest male figure in her life—just pretty much wither away into a weak and frail shell of a man. Cancer is incredibly cruel that way. My father died from an aggressive form of cancer that originated in some unknown organ in his abdomen (doctors were never able to identify which one in biopsies) and it caused inflammation in his abdomen, which is why this rare type of cancer is nicknamed "jelly belly." Having a parent die from abdominal cancer became even more significant to me after I developed chronic pelvic pain issues of my own.

At the beginning of 2002, Guy and I consciously decided to start a family. I went to the doctor for my annual exam and came back with an "abnormal" result on my Pap smear. As I went back into the clinic for the requested repeat exam with the same doctor, she questioned me as to why I was there. When I tried to remind her and said, "It should be in my file," the doctor got snippy with me. My repeat exam was most unpleasant. I felt abused and violated.

That evening, I shared my experience with my husband, and instead of receiving the compassion or empathy I expected, he took my dissatisfaction of the treatment I received at the clinic as a personal attack and failure on his part because the healthcare was provided by his employer. That was the explanation I received from him, after being surprised by his reaction to my uncomfortable experience in the stirrups. Basically, any time I shared my displeasure with the healthcare I received from military institutions constituted a failure on his part. This became a learned lesson that fueled my reluctance to share any of my "negative medical experiences" in the future with him.

Regardless, that "unpleasant Pap" came out normal, and within four months I was pregnant. Guy deployed in June and would be gone for most of the pregnancy. We planned it that way with the hopes he would return in time for the birth and all the fun and bonding that occurs afterward. What I didn't realize was how difficult pregnancy could be as I struggled with morning sickness, which was "all-day sickness." I was incredibly sensitive to smells, like perfumes and cigarette smoke. I also had food aversions to meat, and the sight of raw meat in the grocery store would make me nauseous. Other than that, I felt pretty good until the last trimester, when my body just constantly hurt. My doctor and everyone else told me this was normal—the swollen feet, pressure, heartburn, et cetera.

By this time, Guy was coming home from deployment to a big-bellied wife. I will never forget the excitement I felt inside as the baby kicked to the sound of the horns that blew the day Guy's submarine returned to port. The kicks just about knocked me to the ground. I was pretty sure I was giving birth to a football player, and even though I didn't know that I was having a boy, I was pretty sure he was one.

The last few weeks of the pregnancy were incredibly painful. I began having contractions at 36 weeks gestation but was told they were just Braxton Hicks (sporadic contractions) and get sent home from the hospital with pills to help me sleep and instructed to drink lots of water.

When the baby's due date finally passed, I went back into the hospital with my contractions, five minutes apart, and just wanted the baby out of me. The monitor confirmed I was in full labor, but I wasn't dilated. As I writhed in pain in triage praying to be admitted, a woman smiled being wheeled back into delivery. That was the kind of birth experience I wanted. But no, instead I was taken to have an ultrasound "to see what's going on in there." As it turns out, I suffered from polyhydramnios and cephalopelvic disproportion (CPD). In layman's terms, this is "too much amniotic fluid" and "the baby is too big for mom's pelvis."

In fact, my baby's weight was registering "off the charts." The best the technician could estimate was between nine and thirteen pounds. The largest baby my mom delivered was about eight-and-a-half-pounds, so I was terrified upon hearing these numbers. Interestingly, a study conducted at the Institute of Child Health and published in the journal PLOS ONE linked a baby's birth weight to the "expression of the paternal IGF2 gene." Guy weighed six pounds at birth and was born one month premature, so he probably would have been around ten pounds full term. Family lore tells of a great aunt on his side who was born weighing thirteen pounds. My body hurts just thinking about that. Anyway, I was not going to be delivering my baby with my midwife, as I planned, but was going to be cut open instead. At the time, all I could think about was both of us surviving. My baby was trying to come out for weeks and couldn't, and I felt as if my pelvis was going to snap in half from all the pressure. While a surgeon was lined up, I was sent home with sleeping pills yet again and instructed to return to the hospital at 6:00 a.m. the next morning for surgery.

As one can imagine, I did not get much sleep that night. I had already been sleeping in my husband's recliner for weeks because I was so uncomfortable and couldn't lay down flat or get back up without assistance. My feet had to stay elevated because of the edema, and Guy still had to sleep and go to work during the weeks prior to delivery. Regardless, my husband was amazing, as he would rub my legs (that were more like tree trunks) and massage my feet. You couldn't even recognize my toes because they were so swollen. I was miserable.

The next morning was an adventure as I met my surgeon. I remember him inspecting my abdomen and saying, "Oh, wow." I asked him what he seemed so surprised about, and he said that my uterus expanded up over my pelvic bone. He said usually with cesareans, a doctor had to feel where the bone was and draw a line on the patient where the incision needed to be, but he said that my body was literally saying, "Cut here." He never saw anything so pronounced before.

There were more "surprises" in the operating room as the anesthesiologist was administering my spinal block. It is incredibly difficult when you can't arch your back when you are carrying such a heavy load upfront, and the anesthesiologist must have stabbed me half a dozen times before the needle was inserted properly. The real fun began during the surgery, as my uterus was cut open and all the excess amniotic fluid came pouring out. There were apparently two "saddlebags" on either side of me to catch these bodily liquids, but there was so much fluid that the bags overflowed, and they spilled out onto the operating room floor. The surgeons and nurses were wearing it on their garments too. This was another instance where I heard the words, "Oh, wow."

The sensation of being awake while someone is playing around with your insides is somewhat indescribable. I could feel some tugging as doctors pulled my son out of me, but there was no pain and no excitement; it was as if I was hearing the procedure happen from another room, since there was a curtain drawn up. I was laying on a table with my arms bound with needles and tubes, and I was breathing through an oxygen mask.

Then suddenly, I heard a loud cry that pierced my heart. It was my son, Billy, screaming. He weighed just over five kilograms, or eleven pounds. He was taken to the neonatal intensive care unit (NICU) for observation for a couple of days, which was standard for all babies born over ten pounds delivered via c-section to monitor glucose levels and aspiration.

I don't remember getting sewn back up or being wheeled into my recovery suite. However, I will never forget waking up alone to the most horrific pain I have ever experienced. The anesthesia had worn off and I was trying to ring a nurse and figure out how to get some pain medication because my stomach and privates felt like they were on fire. However, they weren't just burning— it felt like they were pressed up against a red-hot burner on a stove and I couldn't do anything to move away from it or stop the sensation. I was pushing the button, scream- ing and crying to get anyone's attention. Finally, a nurse came in and said that my machine already dispensed the adequate amount of medication and promised I should feel better soon. After fifteen minutes, I was still in pain. The nurse asked me questions, but at this point I couldn't speak because the pain was so severe that I could barely breathe. My nose was plugged up from crying, but I couldn't even blow my nose because you need your abdominal muscles to do that. After over half an hour of playing with Percocet, I was introduced to an amazing drug called Dilaudid that was injected into my thigh and took the pain away almost instantly.

To keep a long story as short as possible, I spent five days in the hospital learning to walk and go to the bath- room again. Since the skin around my stomach was so over-stretched from my pregnancy, I had to wear a binder around my abdomen to prevent my skin from hanging and reopening my incision. Normally, a person recovering from surgery would be instructed to get plenty of rest and not to lift anything over ten pounds, and yes, I was told that, too. However, when your baby weighs eleven pounds and is waking up every two hours to be fed, that just isn't going to happen. I can honestly say I don't remember a whole lot about the first six months of my son's life. Six weeks after his birth, my husband's submarine went into drydock at the Portsmouth Naval Shipyard in Kittery, Maine, and so we moved. Guy rode the submarine up there and I somehow managed to drive our Jeep Grand Cherokee—with my son in a car seat—along with all of the household belongings I could, so that we could live in a hotel until we could find housing. Unfortunately, there was no officer housing available on base, so we ended up renting a two-bedroom apartment attached to someone's garage in town. I honestly have no idea how I managed to make that move all by myself less than two months after delivering a baby via c-section. I know my son wasn't even two months old because I have photos celebrating his first Easter in the hotel room.

Sadly, I spent most of those first six months as a new mom recovering from surgery alone and miserable. We just moved, we weren't living on base, I had no friends close by, my family was over 2,700 miles away, and my husband, who initially promised he would be more available to help once the boat was in drydock, ended up working even more. Apparently, the command decided to keep the galley open, and there was an issue with the boat's inventory that required an audit, and then he even served as acting executive officer for a time.

Meanwhile, our house was never completely unpacked in the six months we lived there. The medical clinic on base had no real OB-GYN care for post-cesarean moms, and after developing mastitis, I was given bad information and ended up in the emergency room of the local hospital with an abscess and high fever. The pain was so bad that I was vomiting, and I couldn't lift my arm. Upon returning from the emergency room, Guy was getting dressed in his uniform to march in the local Memorial Day parade, as I was camped out by the toilet, vomiting. This is what the Navy calls "mando fun," or mandatory fun. As my husband explained it, he couldn't get out of the parade because he was the public relations officer, so he had no choice but to march in the parade. I questioned where the line of common sense in military duty and duty to family crossed. Being that we were new to the area, been in the house about a month at that point, I was very much removed from any support of the military base over 30 miles away. Our ship's ombudsman didn't even make the move. For all the propaganda about military community "taking care of their own," I felt very much like a military dependent, who had been cast aside in her time of need, even after she had stepped up and contributed to support, serving as the President of the Family Support Group during deployment because the position had to be filled in order for family members to receive updates. It appeared that this parade was a bigger priority than mine or my baby's wellbeing.

The following month, this issue resurfaced as we flew to Maryland for the wedding of some good friends we made in Connecticut. In fact, I met my friend Kelly in a base support group, and her fiancé was an officer on another submarine in the squadron. Kelly was incredibly supportive during my pregnancy while our men were out to sea. Besides me and my husband, Kelly was the first person to hold our son after he was born, and it was extremely important to me to be at her wedding at the U.S. Naval Academy Chapel. Kelly and her fiancé asked Guy to be in the wedding as part of the sword arch. The night of the dress rehearsal, I started to feel unwell and developed a fever, and then I started to feel nauseous and went to the emergency room near the hotel. The breast infection returned and required another round of antibiotics. Sadly, I did not get to attend Kelly's wedding and spent the day miserable in the hotel room with Billy, alone, while Guy attended the wedding and reception. Flying home wasn't fun either, as Billy did not inherit my love of travel, crying the entire flight and developing an ear infection. The trip was truly unbelievable, which is why in August, when we were scheduled to fly back home to Idaho for all of our relatives to meet our little man, and Guy informed me that his liberty chit was not approved, I was not willing to make that long, cross-country flight home with a baby all by myself. I was exhausted. At this point, Billy was sleeping only four to six hours at a time, but I felt like I needed him to sleep for forty-six hours. Prolonged sleep deprivation is truly an insidious form of torture.

I recall the conversations I had with Guy about my hesitancy making the trip alone but felt the pressure because family from nearby states already made plans to meet Billy, so I had to make the trip happen. I voiced my concerns about flying cross-country; spending eight to ten hours on airplanes feeding, changing diapers, sleeping; and having to carry on all the baby necessities by myself. Most of those concerns were ameliorated when I had the idea of driving cross-country, where I would have the ability to pull over and do whatever needed to be done whenever it needed to be done, in privacy. There would be no chance of constant crying disturbing the other passengers or chances for developing ear infections like our first airplane experience. I called my mother to see if she would be up for flying out and helping me make this cross-country road trip. She and I made previous road trips together, as I think I inherited my "travel bug" from her. I was grateful that she agreed to help. After making the drive from New Hampshire out to Idaho, which took about a week, I came to realize that I didn't take into consideration the fact that I would be driving the entire eight hours every day and getting up to do the late-night feedings or changings. Taking care of a six-month-old in middle of the night was not conducive to driving eight hours a day for several consecutive days. By the time I got to Idaho, I was exhausted. But I figured I would get caught up on some sleep because all these family members, whom I made the drive for, would be fighting over the baby they came to meet. Unfortunately, we all know how it is—if the baby needs to be fed or changed, Mom usually gets the baby back.

Staying with Guy's side of the family, the house has a revolving door, it was always a busy and noisy house, with people coming and going. Billy was not getting his naps and was crying more than usual. I recall mentioning the noise level to the family and everyone laughed and said, "He will get used to it," and gave advice like, "You should run the vacuum cleaner when he's napping so he can learn to sleep through noise." I know everyone has advice on what new moms should do, but I was trying to follow the "sleep when baby sleeps" advice because if I vacuumed when he slept, I would never get any sleep, which was something I so desperately needed in order to heal.

The road trip back to New Hampshire after the visit was just as exhausting and stressful. I vomited the moment I walked into the house straight up to the bathroom. I swore I was never going to make that journey again with an infant. It was just too much, and honestly, at that point, I was never going to have another child.

The fun, however, was not over, as three months later we were moving again; this time to the Washington, D.C., area, where Guy would have a five-year shore duty and "be around the house more to help." Unfortunately, we came to realize that Billy, who was almost one-year old at this point, only bonded with me and I was the only one who could soothe him. Since he was now strictly bottle-fed, we looked at putting him in daycare so that I could have the freedom to go back to school or work, and Billy could learn to deal with mommy separation. But unfortunately, as what usually happens with children when they first enter daycare, I was getting calls almost weekly, to come pick him up because of a rash, a fever, or a snotty nose.

The weekend of the fourth of July, we planned to go to Atlantic City for a family vacation with some of Guy's co-workers. The day before we were scheduled to leave, I got a call from the daycare letting me know that Billy had pink eye and I needed to get him. I picked him up, took him to the doctor, got a prescription, and was told that Billy would be contagious for three to seven days depending on when his eyes cleared up. I mentioned we were planning to go on vacation, and the pediatrician said that would not be wise since Conjunctivitis is highly contagious, and we had to be mindful about washing hands all the time and not spreading the infection on to others. Billy could even contaminate a hotel room by touching things. When I informed Guy about this, he became frustrated due to the fact that there was a $100, non-refundable deposit on our hotel room. Guy suggested Billy and I could just stay in the room. Billy had a fever and goopy eyes, and I recall saying I would rather stay at home, where we had everything that we might need to soothe him. I had flashbacks of when I had a fever in the hotel room in Maryland a year before and how I felt. In the end, I stayed home to take care of Billy alone, and Guy went off to Atlantic City with his friends.

I had a horrible holiday weekend. Aside from having a baby with a fever and trying to put antibiotics in a one-year-old's eyes, my back seized up on me either while I was picking Billy up or putting him in his crib, and I was in horrendous pain. I ended up laying on the floor waiting for the spasm to subside. This wasn't the first time that something like that happened to me, but it was one of the worst instances in a while. So much so, that I took some Vicodin to help with the pain. By the end of the weekend, I downed the entire bottle and just wanted to sleep for eternity, but then I thought, who would take care of Billy? It certainly wasn't going to be his father, who chose to play in Atlantic City. I cried and went into the bathroom and made myself throw up. When Guy did get home, I confided in him what I did, and he insisted I go to the doctor and get help because something was seriously wrong with me.

Instantly, I was diagnosed as having post-partum depression, so I was referred to a psychiatrist, who prescribed me a selective serotonin reuptake inhibitor (SSRI) antidepressant. Looking back, and knowing what I know now, this was not helpful because the side effects of antidepressants are insomnia, headaches, nausea, and reduced sexual desire, which were all things I already suffered from. However, what did help was the referral to the cognitive-behavioral therapist, who got me talking about everything that happened over the last couple of years. She said that there wasn't anything wrong with me, and that what I was feeling was perfectly normal considering everything I went through. I was "soldiering on" for far too long, not dealing with my feelings of grief, not having the positive birth experience that I expected, and the isolation and loneliness of the military lifestyle. The constant keeping busy and moving, and not dealing with these feelings of loss and grief coupled by the exhaustion had fueled my depression. It wasn't just post-partum hormones.

Chapter 3:

It's Going to Be Different This Time

*"You gain strength, courage and confidence
by every experience in which you stop
to look fear in the face. You must do
the thing you think you cannot do."*
– Eleanor Roosevelt, *You Learn by Living: Eleven Keys
for a More Fulfilling Life (1960)*

The surgeon who performed my c-section originally told me that it would take about two years for my body to completely heal in order to safely become pregnant again. I was deathly afraid of delivering another child, and this was my initial aversion to having sex with my husband. In my mind, there was no way to ensure my safety. I truly believed if I got pregnant again, I was going to die.

Once the two-year-mark passed though, I began to feel better. I was also more settled in our new home in Virginia; was taking college courses online; doing genealogy research; and joined two volunteer service organizations, the Daughters of the American Revolution and the Military Spouses Residency Relief Act Coalition. That following summer, Billy and I took a road trip and visited a friend of mine living in Austin, Texas. She had a daughter, who was a few months younger than Billy, and she just had another baby. When I saw how Billy interacted with Buffy—walking, talking, and playing with her—I realized what an amazing big brother he would be, and I felt as if I needed to get over my fear of pregnancy. I told myself that I was wiser and would be prepared this time. I knew what to expect and depression was not going to happen again.

When I came home from that trip, I told Guy about the epiphany I had and that I'd made peace with what happened before, and I wanted to have another baby. This time, I wanted to have a girl. Guy made no promises about the girl part, but within that first month, I was pregnant with our second child.

My second pregnancy did feel completely different than my first one. I had some morning sickness but didn't experience the all-day stuff as I did before. I also didn't experience the food aversions I had while pregnant with Billy. In fact, I craved meat, especially steak. The military health clinic in Virginia had its own OB-GYN staff and was associated with the military hospital that had labor and delivery. They had records of my previous birth experience and assured me that they were closely monitoring my situation to prevent a repeat experience. Our goal was for a vaginal birth after cesarean (VBAC). Everything seemed to be on par for the perfect "normal pregnancy experience." Guy and I flew back home to Idaho for Christmas that year, and my doctor recommended I get a flu shot before I traveled, as it was anticipated to be a bad flu season. I never had a flu shot before and never got the flu, so I wasn't keen on the idea. Guy said he gets flu vaccinations all the time being military and "it's not a big deal." My doctor persisted and, while acknowledging it was my choice, she insisted.

So, I got the flu shot, and it was my first, and last, flu shot to date. Getting a flu shot temporarily compromises your immune system to form the antibodies. The flu strain for Virginia was likely not the same strain one would be exposed to in Idaho, or by any sick passenger on an airplane. Out of the three of us flying, guess who got the flu? Yup, that would be me—the one who got the flu shot, the one who was pregnant and was restricted on what medications she could take. On the flight home, my eardrum ruptured, and I ended up going to the emergency room and receiving antibiotics. The antibiotics resulted in a subsequent yeast infection, a recurring, unpleasant experience for the remainder of my pregnancy.

I chose to see a different OB-GYN after returning from the holiday, but my new doctor was then transferred to another duty station. My third doctor later determined that I was likely going to require another cesarean section due to my size and the yeast infection issue, so I was referred to doctor number four, who was also pregnant. She planned to do my surgery and agreed to address my issue of the excess skin that hung off my abdomen from my first pregnancy. This procedure is referred to as a "c-tuck," a cesarean with tummy tuck. In doing this, I hoped to avoid the weight of the over-stretched skin pulling on my incision and having to wear an uncomfortable binder again. Unfortunately, my doctor went into labor before I did, and I was assigned as a patient to my fifth doctor. He was a colonel and reputed as one of the best surgeons at the hospital.

Many women shared horror stories regarding their birth experiences at this hospital, and the main piece of advice I read was, "If they ask you if it is okay to have an intern in the operating room, do it. Just insist that the intern can't do anything, only observe." Doctors tend to be meticulous and do a better job when an intern is in the room watching their every move, and as luck would have it, on the morning of my scheduled c-section I was asked if it would be all right if an intern observed during my operation. Although I was still nervous about the operation, I felt a bit better that this surgeon would be extra attentive with an intern watching him, I responded as I was advised to by my colleagues.

The surgery appeared to be going well and my daughter was born relatively quickly. Guy went with her and to complete some paperwork while the doctor was closing me up; unfortunately, he did not do the "c-tuck" as planned. I remember him instructing the intern on how to do the stitches and then things began to fade. I woke up in a recovery room and remember the staff talking to me, only for my vision to go fuzzy and seeing double. The nurses asked me to describe how I was feeling. I recall one nurse saying that my vitals weren't remaining steady.

Then suddenly, I started to experience contractions. They were intermittent, but it was strange because I didn't have any contractions prior to the surgery, and I didn't recall having that experience after Billy was born. Why was I having contractions when I was no longer pregnant? Uterine contractions following a surgery are extremely uncomfortable. I did my best to bear down while tied down by IV tubes and the wires from the monitoring equipment. I then remember being wheeled into another room, where doctors and staff were attempting to determine the cause of my increased heart rate and blood pressure issues. At this point, I recall Guy being in the room and getting frustrated with the doctors because they kept giving me more units of blood, but nothing was changing, and no one could seem to get an ultrasound machine to the room to get an idea of what was going on inside my body. Guy was pretty sure I had internal bleeding, because his father had died from injuries suffered in an automobile accident a few years prior. He was frustrated by the lack of action that was occurring in the room because the colonel insisted everything was normal when he closed me up. After some tests, they confirmed I had internal bleeding and I was wheeled back into the operating room, this time completely under anesthesia, and would spend the next two days in the intensive care unit (ICU) of the hospital recovering.

Yet again, this was not the birth experience I planned or hoped for. Guy was only able to get every other day off from work, but luckily my mom flew out to help with Billy for that first week. I spent five days at that hospital, and it was the most surreal experience. While in the ICU, I had limited visitation and mobility. I had an IV in one arm while my other arm was elevated because the IV was originally in that arm but blew out and became swollen. My room was right across from the nurses' station; however, it wasn't always occupied. It was extremely difficult to press a call button or control my medication when I couldn't move either of my arms. I also wasn't capable of yelling loudly after having a breathing tube down my throat. It was extremely frustrating because sometimes the phone in my room would ring and I had no way of answering it, only to find out later that it was the nursery two floors up calling to see if I wanted to nurse my baby. After all my body had been through, it was far too weak, and I never produced milk anyway, but it would have been nice to see and hold my baby.

This was ironic because, with Billy, I couldn't go to the grocery store or be gone for an hour anywhere without my body becoming engorged. I could have fed twins, or even triplets, with my milk production with Billy, but not this time. Without a doubt, this birth experience was different. Once I was stable and moved up to the maternity ward, I received a visit from the La Leche breastfeeding representative, who unwisely asked me if I was breastfeeding my baby. When I responded in the negative, but before I could finish and explain why, the representative cut me off to inform me why I should breastfeed and that it was healthier for my baby. At that point, I broke down and asked her to leave. Breastfeeding became a triggering issue again after I was home. I'm not sure why this was because I didn't particularly enjoy breastfeeding like some women do—I honestly felt like a cow. However, psychologically, the fact that you can't provide for your infant is demoralizing.

The following week or two, apparently some of Guy's friends invited him to go out and play poker, and he said he couldn't because he needed to stay home with me and our daughter. The friend asked, "Why? Do you need to wet nurse the baby?" Although I'm pretty sure this friend had no idea what I went through, I found his comment shameful and demeaning of women regardless. These negative experiences were only the beginning of the physical and emotional distress I experienced following my daughter's delivery. When someone is physically hurting, they are more susceptible to hurt emotionally. Or when someone is emotionally hurting, they are more open to physical pain. It is a vicious cycle.

Chapter 4:

Traveling the Road to Recovery While Navigating the Healthcare System

"And a woman spoke, saying, 'tell us of pain,' and he said: your pain is the breaking of the shell that encloses your understanding. Even as the stone of the fruit must break, that its heart may stand in the sun, so must you know pain."
– Kahlil Gibran, *The Prophet (1923)*

s one can imagine, recovering from an ordeal like this is a process, and luckily, I had family and friends who came out, visited, and helped me for the first couple of weeks afterward. Even though I nearly died, I felt so much better immediately following this delivery than after my first c-section because I felt physically and emotionally supported, and that does make all the difference.

According to statistics reported by the Centers for Disease Control and Prevention's Division of Reproductive Health, the U.S. maternal mortality rate has more than doubled in the last thirty years. Over 700 women die each year from complications due to pregnancy and over fifty thousand women suffer from life-threatening complications. The United States is the only developed country in the world to experience an increase while the global maternal mortality rate has decreased. It is estimated that two-thirds of these complications are preventable, however it appears that our healthcare system is not interested in preventing these complications, only in treating the symptoms. In order to get help in today's healthcare system, most people must first be seen by their primary care provider (PCP) or general practitioner (GP). Then that person refers you to a specialist in whatever area of health the PCP/GP believes the ailment falls under. This makes navigating our healthcare system and getting a proper diagnosis and treatment extremely difficult, especially if your GP isn't educated in your condition.

My physical recovery after the birth of my second child was incredibly slow. Doctors told me to be patient with myself, but I had a job, a house, and a husband and kids to care for, so I needed to get back in the game. In April of 2007, one year after my surgeries, my PCP/GP reported I was "normal." But in June, I went back into the doctor's office complaining of "body aches, fatigue, and headaches" and it was determined to be "allergies."

In December, I went in complaining of "stomach pains," but in my chart my doctor only wrote "cystitis?" I was given a prescription for Nitrofurantoin.

I returned to the clinic in February of 2008 complaining of abdominal pains again, and my patient record quoted, "Patient states has not felt normal since delivery. Thinks she has adhesions. Has had irregular cycles last two months. Has had decreased appetite." After the lab results came back, my PCP diagnosis was, "IBS?" I was prescribed a fiber supplement.

A month later, I was back into the clinic reporting that I was experiencing lower back pain and sciatica. My PCP said I was "normal," but noted that I was, "overweight with possible sacroiliac (SI) joint dysfunction." She recommended physical therapy, and noted, "appears to be piriformis muscle, unless worsen, no urgency."

A week later, I saw a different doctor at the clinic and complained of lower back pain, sciatica, and fatigue. The doctor ordered an x-ray and an ultrasound of my pelvis. However, when I called to make the appointment at the military hospital, the wait was four to six weeks. When I asked about a waitlist, I was told the hospital did not have one. However, I learned that they must leave some slots open for the emergency room. At my husband's suggestion, I decided to spend my next day off from work, during the following week, hanging out in the hospital emergency room to get my x-ray and ultrasound.

That next week, now April of 2008 and one year after I began complaining about my symptoms, my x-ray results said, "normal except mild degeneration in left hip." My ultrasound results said, "uterus size at 10.6 by 6 by 4.2 centimeters, no fibroids, unremarkable." The doctor prescribed methocarbamol, often used to treat muscle spasms and pain, and physical therapy, while putting in an order for an MRI. My follow-up appointment for my MRI results was with my PCP, and she said that my results showed "normal alignment and were unremarkable."

When I confided in her that sex was extremely painful, to the point that I didn't want to engage in sex at all, she said, "You can't deny your husband." Was that her medical opinion or her personal belief? Because if she experienced how much it hurt and how it occasionally caused me to bleed too, she probably would change her mind. But, she then questioned why I had not yet been to physical therapy. When I explained that the orders were on the military base and my work and home were thirty and forty miles away. It was not convenient to drive there two to three times a week around my work schedule and daycare, especially when I felt that physical therapy wasn't addressing the real issue. Still, she gave me some real grief, saying my issues stemmed from obesity and the sex issues were due to a lack of lubrication and I should try a gel. I disagreed with her and told her I had no trouble getting wet or turned on. It was an internal stabbing-like pain during and that the pain remained for a day or two after intercourse. After this appointment, I requested a change of PCP/GP and refused to go to her again, as I felt she neither listened to me nor cared.

In May of 2008, I gave my notice at the travel agency where I worked and instead would help manage the small business my husband started back in February of 2007, while doing the physical therapy sessions as prescribed two to three times a week. These sessions involved core strengthening exercises, pelvic level exercises, deep tissue massage, interferential current therapy, among other therapies. I was also given a prescription for Robaxin and Tylenol. I attended these physical therapy sessions until I was discharged, saying that I received the "maximum benefit" on November 19, 2008. And yet, I felt as if nothing had changed. This was about the time that I started paying out of pocket to see a chiropractor, because military health insurance did not cover chiropractic care for military family members. In fact, even the military service members weren't eligible until 2001 and only then at military hospital locations.

In January of 2009, my children and I all requested a final wellness check-up at the clinic, as Guy was resigning his commission with the Navy. Since our daughter's birth, I had been to over thirty doctor's appointments at this point, not counting the chiropractor. That's an average of over one a month. I was also taking our children to their doctor's appointments, which included well baby check-ups and immunizations. I was also working outside the home that entire time, until I quit my job six months prior to run my husband's business at his urging. The business grew 366 percent within the first year of my involvement. I wasn't just driving it; I was steamrolling it. So you can imagine my surprise when I would later read in our divorce documents that he wrote, "In 2009, after trying to help the Defendant for years through numerous mental and physical issues, and finding the Defendant to be unwilling to take personal responsibility for her welfare, Plaintiff began to lose hope in his ability to help Defendant live an emotionally healthy life and saw that the objects of the marriage were no longer existent." What I came to realize is the way people treat us is a statement of who they are as a human being. The fact is he was not a witness to my pain. I can count the doctors' appointments where he accompanied me on one hand. He was physically and emotionally absent. His priority was his career. Pain alienates us because people naturally try to avoid feeling pain. Even though this pain was caused by our mutual decision to have children, he didn't view this as being ours to work through together. It was apparently mine to work through alone.

As a man, he had the luxury of walking away from any responsibility, while I carried the physical consequences of childbirth. It reminded me of the speech that Elizabeth Cady Stanton gave in 1892 titled, *The Solitude of Self*, when fighting for women's equal rights, she stated, "Whatever the theories may be of woman's dependence on man, in the supreme moments of her life, he cannot bear her burdens. Alone she goes to the gates of death to give life to every man that is born into the world; no one can share her fears, no one can mitigate her pangs; and if her sorrow is greater than she can bear, alone she passes beyond the gates into the vast unknown. From the mountain-tops of Judea long ago, a heavenly voice bade his disciples, "Bear ye one another's burdens"; but humanity has not yet risen to that point of self-sacrifice; and if ever so willing, how few the burdens are that one soul can bear for another!"

It takes great strength to be in pain, especially for an extended length of time. It takes even greater strength to endure the pain and still function as a caregiver and employee. The doctor, who finally diagnosed me, was my witness after my surgery when she said, "I don't know how you were functioning." That is all the proof and validation I needed to know, in that I persevered and got the job done despite my condition.

Like my ex-husband, doctors are critical thinkers, who are comfortable making decisions without all the facts. This is a fantastic skill to have, if you need to make quick decisions. However, if you are a patient and have a doctor, who doesn't listen to you attentively, they are not necessarily going to make the best decisions for you and your specific situation. Their decision will be based on their past patients and their past experiences. I had several doctors, who did not listen well. I had some doctors, who just didn't know what was wrong, because they perhaps were not educated with the conditions that I had, primarily adenomyosis and diastasis recti. This was the true tragedy.

The doctor, who diagnosed me in 2015 as having adenomyosis, informed me that the ultrasound conducted in April of 2008 stated that my uterus size was 10.6 by 6 by 4.2 centimeters. No one doctor, who viewed that report, recognized that as being slightly enlarged. The average woman's uterus is 7.6 by 4.5 by 3 centimeters.

Why does the size of the uterus matter, you might be asking? One way that the uterine disease adenomyosis can be recognized is through use of imaging and seeing characteristics of the disease, such as an enlarged size or lack of definition between the two main layers of the uterus, the endometrium and myometrium. A normal uterus shows distinct layers. Adenomyosis is the buildup of endometrial cells in the myometrium. The endometrium is the inner layer that sheds each month with the menstrual cycle. The myometrium is the uterine muscle tissue. When the endometrial cells invade or get implanted in the myometrium, they can get trapped. During menstruation, they will respond to hormonal stimulation and bleed, but the blood will also get trapped. With each month, the cells replicate, and more fluid gets trapped, and the uterus expands. With the pressure of the fluid buildup, the muscle will contract attempting to expel it. Sometimes it is successful. I experienced spotting or even an occasional "second monthly period."

When I shared with my husband that I would notice this "second period," he minimized my concern saying that the only coincidence between having sex and bleeding after was merely because "you get horny right before your period." There is nothing about adenomyosis that makes a woman "horny."

Symptoms of adenomyosis include, but are not limited to, painful and prolonged menstruation, and with the increased blood loss, typically anemia and fatigue follow. Infertility, painful intercourse, and depression are also common. Sadly, not much is known about this relatively common disease. However, statistics have shown that eighty percent of women with adenomyosis also have other uterine lesions, such as fibroid tumors and seventy percent of women with adenomyosis also have endometriosis. With inflammation being at the root of most diseases, the increased fluid buildup of adenomyosis causing pressure and an enlarged uterus, this can lead to a host of other problems like Pelvic Inflammatory Disease and Pelvic Congestion Syndrome.

Adenomyosis is described by the medical community as being a common condition, estimating that one in ten women will develop it, although they aren't sure what exactly causes it. There appears to be a higher instance with women, whom have endured a trauma to the uterus, whether it be via c-section, enlarged baby or rape. It is often misdiagnosed, but it is considered a benign (non-life threatening) disease. Whether this is considered life-threatening or not, it certainly kills a woman's quality of life, and indirectly can affect her husband's and children's lives as well.

In the case of my friend Maria, she has suffered pain from" the first day of her first menstrual period at the age of fourteen." In her book, *Why Can't Anyone Help Me? The Nightmare of Adenomyosis*, Maria Yeager tells of her seventeen-year struggle to receive a diagnosis and become "cured." I use quotes when saying cured because the only known "cure" for adenomyosis is a hysterectomy, or removal of the organ.

Considering one in ten women may have the disease and this is the only known cure—the removal of her reproductive organ—I can't help but wonder how a man would feel if these were the odds he faced. There is a lot of grief and shame associated with losing your reproductive organs and to know that this is currently the only way to live a pain-free life is pitiful beyond words. Maria had her hysterectomy in 2007, and it is thanks to her books and online Adenomyosis Fighters support group that I suspected adenomyosis for myself, before any doctor ever used the term with me. Her willingness to share her story to help others was invaluable to me. She and I agreed in a recent phone conversation that we wouldn't wish "even our worst enemy to endure the years of pain and mistreatment we have been through." We feel as if the "care" in healthcare is truly lacking.

In her book, *Daring Greatly: How the Courage to Be Vulnerable Transforms the Way We Live, Love, Parent and Lead*, Brené Brown says, "If we can share our story with someone who responds with empathy and understanding, shame can't survive." This perfectly describes why Maria has written her books and encouraged me to finish mine, because not only does it allow us to help heal others, but it also helps us to heal ourselves on another level.

I share this background with you so that you understand that your chronic pelvic pain is likely caused by some injury or event that set the wheels in motion. My injury occurred during my first pregnancy, and then was compounded in the second pregnancy. Normally, when an injury occurs, the body has a way of healing itself. But when it can't heal itself properly, it needs active assistance. If the body doesn't get the help it needs, it goes into "survival mode" and does whatever it can to keep running and sends off warning alerts in the form of pain. Like any machine, the body will start slowing down or even shut off some systems it deems less essential. Often, one can become distracted by these "shut-downs" and not see the underlying cause that needs to be addressed. This becomes particularly difficult when you are in chronic pain, because pain is a huge distractor.

In the chapters that follow, I will discuss several root causes of chronic pelvic pain and their distractors. I will also outline some ways that you can feel safe and in control of your body. These are simple ways that just require breaking old habits, but after some practice and patience will become rituals in your daily life. These rituals will get you H-E-A-L-E-D, in the realms of Hope, Exercise, Amor/Heart, Lullaby/Sleep, Environment, and Diet.

Chapter 5:

Hope Sparks a Willingness to Act

"Strength does not come from physical capacity. It comes from an indomitable will."
– Mahatma Gandhi

In taking the course on Compassion Cultivation Training, developed at Stanford University, I have learned that there are a few steps for a person to take in order to actively provide support when one is suffering.

First, there needs to be a recognition or awareness of the suffering.

Then one must feel concern and have a desire to relieve the suffering.

The next step is believing that you can do something and make a difference.

And the fourth step is having the willingness to act.

I was fully aware of my pain, and I was far beyond concerned and desiring relief. Where I kept getting stuck was believing that the pain could be eliminated. I would walk into each doctor's appointment hoping for answers but walk out feeling like I was physically and emotionally beat up.

What I realized after seeing over a dozen different doctors, none of whom found anything of significance physically, was that they trusted the technology over their patients and implied that the pain was imaginary. When medical testing fails to find a plausible cause for a person's pain, it must be mindset. This kind of reasoning assumes that our current medical technology can detect any and all possible organic causes of pain, even though pain is a sensation; a feeling. It can't appear in bloodwork or an ultrasound. And being that imaging technology was incapable of showing the full extent of my pelvic adhesions, or that a nerve injury during surgery can lead to chronic pain, we really need to learn to trust our instincts more. The idea that I was somehow fabricating my pain scared me even more than the pain did. I seriously considered the theory for a moment but then I found the concept was even more crazy making. I concluded that doctors, when they can't come up with the answer, instead of just saying

"I don't know" will say "there is nothing wrong with you." To me this appears to be all ego, as we expect doctors to know everything, and they in return give us that impression. The truth is, they are human, just like us and they aren't perfect. They can get things wrong and with me, they did, for several years, because I had multiple conditions and they didn't "see" any of them. No one likes to admit a failure, however, to suggest or even convince a patient that her struggles are concocted or are inconsequential because "it's not cancer," is vicious. No one should feel that the only way they can be taken seriously is to hope they receive a cancer diagnosis.

I had been trying the "mind over matter" and bullying myself through the pain to survive and do everything I had been doing as a wife, a mother and a businesswoman, without taking much pain medication for years. Looking back with a clear perspective, this was all wrong. The mental and physical aspects of our bodies are not separate entities but are very much intertwined and co-dependent. My mind knew that my body was injured, but the doctors were not listening to me, and instead of listening to my intuition I was believing these people with their PHDs knew more than I did. After a decade of trying to diagnose the source of my pain, which several doctors told me to stop searching WebMD, because I was making myself hysterical, I had nothing. No proof, no evidence. No answers.

But with Guy no longer in the military, I wasn't limited to just seeing military doctors anymore, which was wonderful. However, I was starting all over again on my quest for answers, trying to find doctors who were accepting new clients, who accepted his government insurance, and listened to my concerns. I needed a doctor to find some legitimate evidence of my issues so that they could refer me to a specialist in order to be cured of whatever was causing my pain. At the same time, I had a first grader and a child at a daycare, all while I was trying to manage my husband's business from home. I denied myself the pain medications so my mind could stay sharp working numbers all day, and I could drive my kids to their meetings and practices without being "under the influence" of opioids. Guy worked in Washington, DC and left the house by 5am and usually wasn't home until 7pm or sometimes later. He unfortunately wasn't available most of the time to help with the home or his business.

To keep the rest of my personal story as brief as possible, over the next five years I would see a new doctor (GP) each year and have a minimum of one annual exam, always mentioning my concerns/symptoms. The government insurance changed almost annually, from GEHA to Aetna to United Healthcare and then to Anthem. This also brought about its own challenges in my quest for a doctor who could give me a diagnosis, because not all doctors accept all insurance policies.

However, one GP, whom I saw in April of 2014, also noticed my inflammation and obesity, and observed the hardness of my abdomen and requested an ultrasound of my pelvis. This appointment was the direct result after I experienced a "tearing" feeling from doing some exercises from a workout video that one of my husband's friends had produced. In the appointment, I really pressed the issue of possible scar tissue/adhesions because the tear I felt resembled Velcro being ripped up my entire left side, from the hip bone to lower ribcage. It was incredibly painful to the point that it caused me to vomit. The doctor said that nothing was evident in the scan to indicate adhesions. There were no fibroids or abnormalities of the uterus, but that didn't mean there wasn't something going on inside. She then ended the conversation with, "Even if there is something inside, it's not like its cancer. It will go away with menopause." This was the first time that a doctor ever hinted at what I would later learn is called adenomyosis. When I asked if there was a way to find out if the problem was in my uterus, she said there was no evidence to warrant such a procedure and insurance wouldn't therefore cover such an invasive, exploratory procedure. Looking back, I think this doctor believed I was in pain, she considered adenomyosis as a possibility, but had no physical evidence to act on, so therefore felt she could do nothing else for me. According to her there wasn't any evidence of anything even for a referral.

After coming home from this appointment, in which I was writhing in pain from the transvaginal ultrasound, I shared this information with Guy, who at this point appeared completely checked out of attempting to understand anything I tried to explain as to why yet another doctor's appointment resulted in a dead end. His lack of compassion and understanding was substantiated in the later divorce documents, when he stated, "In 2014, Defendant received poor medical advice that waiting for menopause, rather than undergoing surgery, would help alleviate her severe internal pain. Without consulting Plaintiff, Defendant accepted this recommendation and did not seek additional advice. This course of action would have essentially eliminated any quality physical relations for over fifteen years. Plaintiff, unaware of this course of action, continued to feel continuously rejected due to the lack of any physical intimacy."

To read this was extremely infuriating, as, first, he wasn't at that doctor's appointment—or any of my doctor's appointments for that matter—over the past eight years. According to the doctor, nothing was evident in that scan. Like everything before, it was deemed "unremarkable." I wasn't offered any surgical procedure.

What I also found interesting to note was that Guy was predicting my date for menopause to occur at age fifty-eight in the year 2029, while the average age for menopause in women is between forty-eight to fifty-five. Being that my mother had reached menopause naturally at fifty-years-old, and in fact my ovaries shriveled up shortly after the hysterectomy at age forty-eight, this confirms for me that he really didn't try to understand my medical issues, or understand anything about menopause or women's health issues in general. It seemed all he really wanted to blame me for were his own personal fears and insecurities about sex and his "questioning his manhood," as he put it. I understand he was frustrated but taking it out on the patient is like blaming a person, who gets hit by a car while she is in the crosswalk with a green light, and then getting upset with her for the delay in traffic because she has injuries that prevent her from moving. It's unfortunate that the people stuck in traffic are inconvenienced, but at least they aren't the ones laying on the asphalt bleeding.

Chapter 6:

Exercise—The Second Leg

*"I have been impressed with the urgency of
doing. Knowing is not enough; We must apply.
Being willing is not enough; We must do."*
– Leonardo da Vinci

After my hysterectomy in 2015, I worked with a personal trainer who taught me to do targeted stretching and incorporated exercises for me that were intended to strengthen my core and hips using movement progressions primarily among the abdominals, obliques, and hip flexors. Walking and yoga (or Qigong, or Tai Chi) are wonderful, low-impact ways to get in some exercise without overtaxing your sympathetic nervous system, which is what regulates your adrenals and sets off that whole "fight or flight," chronic pain, vicious cycle rabbit hole we don't want to go down. Slow and steady wins the race. If someone tells you that you need to do cardio and lift kettlebells because yoga isn't real exercise, you can tell him that that may work for him, but it will likely cause you injury and pain. Listen to your body. An infant doesn't go from crawling to running and neither should you when you are babying an injury. The phrase "no pain, no gain" is a bully phrase. Consistency and patience with specific mind-body practices are far more effective and provide more rapid relief with minimal side effects. Start out slowly at fifteen minutes and progress from there. Let your body be your coach.

When it comes to women's pelvic muscles, your hips should be strong enough to hold your pelvis and spine in place, but not so tight that it pulls other muscles and joints out of alignment. Chronic tightness in the hips can lead to pain and injury, such as in your knees and lower back. After months and years of seeing chiropractors and physical therapists, I have found that most agree that tight hips are typically caused by core dysfunction, weak legs (particularly in the glutes and hamstrings), weak hip flexors, and incorrect seated posture. My chiropractor was puzzled as to why I continued to show little to no improvement in maintaining alignment after all the work he knew I was putting in to try and recover. My core abdominal muscles were still weak, and it was extremely frustrating.

As I mentioned earlier, my son was born at just over five kilograms or eleven pounds. While pregnant, I carried him completely out front and later learned that my linea alba, the ligament that holds the right and left abdominal muscle walls together had been overextended during pregnancy. This separation of the abdominal muscles is called a diastasis, and this wasn't discovered by doctors until two years after I had my hysterectomy, and fifteen years after he was born, because I developed a ventral hernia. Abdominal separation is normal after childbirth, the average gap after recovery is around two centimeters. I had a seven-centimeter gap. I was trying to use muscles that were incapable of functioning in their condition.

Diastasis of the recti abdominus muscles is often seen in women, who carry twins, which is why doctors in Virginia didn't consider it for me, because I never had twins. However, my one child, who was the size of twins was born in a Connecticut hospital in the military healthcare system, so the Commonwealth of Virginia didn't have it on their database. When I think about the multiple times I moved, carried and lifted my children, boxes, groceries, etc. traveling across country with all that luggage, and just all of the things moms will do in the span of fifteen years, and did all of it without my core abdominal muscles attached and functioning properly. Well, it really explains all of those muscle cramps and back spasms and pain that I endured. And then add the pain of adenomyosis to the equation and it's a wonder I accomplished anything at all, to be honest.

In her book, *Diastasis Recti: The Whole-Body Solution to Abdominal Weakness and Separation*, Katy Bowman describes, "The linea alba, like the elastic in your socks, is pretty resilient. However, there is a point at which the stretch is in the wrong direction, too frequent, held too long, or all three. In this case, the sock elastic is shot. Your linea alba has a threshold of deformation before it gives into the load and deforms permanently." She also states that the linea alba is indirectly connected to everything, as almost all motions of the body are associated with our central core. Just stand for a moment and lift your arms over your head and stretch reaching up on your toes as if you are reaching for the ceiling. Can you feel those abdominal muscles engaging? The crazy thing was that I couldn't. I had asked my personal trainer many times, "Am I doing this exercise right, because I can't feel it." It all makes so much sense in retrospect. And yes, it really upsets me that no one could see why, when it was there the whole time, and I had been asking for help for over a decade.

The diastasis was ultimately discovered because I had developed a hernia. The gap in my abdominal muscles was just above the navel or umbilicus. The hernia likely occurred because after the hysterectomy, my big, old uterus wasn't there to plug the hole, so to speak. It was essentially big enough to block the gap and prevent other things, like my intestines, from falling out.

I had noticed when I exercised that I would sometimes feel nauseous after doing crunches or planks. And downward facing dog, which is supposed to be a relaxing yoga pose, was often not comfortable for me, due to its gravitational pressure of being in an inverted position. I would occasionally say something to my trainer about feeling queasy. I'd take a short break, catch my breath or grab a drink of water., but we figured it was just from being out of shape and then I would just push through it.

Having an exercise accountability buddy can be a wonderful thing. They can keep you motivated and focused. However, one hurdle I experienced in exercising with others is that some people see it as a competition and feel the need to "measure" progress. I have personally never been one for assigning numbers and "values" to things. When it came to work with the medicine ball, for example, I would use the "little blue one" first and then advance to the "medium sized green one." I had no idea how much they weighed and if someone told me or I read it, I honestly wouldn't remember. Don't misunderstand me, exercising with others can be fun and make the time go by more quickly, but it needs to be with the right people, who are willing to work at your pace and be encouraging with where you are, not where they think you should be. For example, if you are with someone who judges and won't go to a yoga class with you because you are not at "his level" then that is not supportive. True yogis will support everyone at whatever level they are at and know how to adapt poses for themselves in any class situation, especially if they are at the high level they claim to be. All yoga sessions begin with a greeting, an intention and a leave-taking; Namaskaram. This gesture is an acknowledgement of the soul of one for the soul of another and is a sign of respect. If you find you have an exercise partner, or an instructor, or anyone for that matter, who does not respect where you are in your practice then you can and should wish them well on their practice and find a more supportive environment. Yes, I had an unsupportive yoga partner experience. Namaste.

In my initial physical therapy sessions, I would get out of breath relatively quickly without getting my heart rate up very high. I also did not like to do "hot yoga" because I had trouble with breathing and felt as if I might pass out. I would later learn that my pelvic congestion issues affected my diaphragm. The diaphragm and the pelvic floor muscles have a core function relationship, so if one is out of balance, the other will not function properly due to pressure. With adenomyosis and its enlarged uterus, the pressure increased. It is this pressure which causes most pregnant women in the last trimester to have issues with their breathing.

Doing yoga and learning diaphragmatic breathing, focusing on the shift from lungs to abdominal breathing, using slow and long deep exhalations conditions the muscles and organs that they can receive their oxygen and nutrients in a "rest and digest" mode. This is a much better environment, as opposed to the "fight or flight" mode of cardio. This is what is termed in the medical community as "Hacking the Vagus Nerve." The vagus nerve is an instrumental part of the parasympathetic nervous system, which supports all function of the heart, lungs and digestion. This is the area of our basic human needs, of air and food, and how our body processes it. In order to feel safe, we need to establish a calm, safe space in which to practice.

Physical safety is a very strong survival instinct, identified in American psychologist Abraham Maslow's *Hierarchy of Needs* (1943). In his ordered hierarchy, without meeting the basic human needs at the bottom of the pyramid, one cannot achieve the human potential and self-actualization at the top of the pyramid. At the base of the pyramid are the basic human needs at an infant state; eat, poop, sleep, breathe, et cetera. This is really what we need to look at, because if we aren't doing this properly, then how can we live a happy, fulfilling life at the top of Maslow's pyramid?

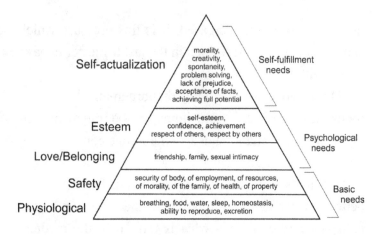

When we consider that the goal of exercise is simply to get the body moving, blood flowing, oxygen circulating, so as to create some energy, lose some weight, gain some muscle or gain some flexibility, it is a fact that all of this can be achieved without stressing the body.

One website and program that I found most informative, to the point of being almost invaluable was at www.nataliehodson.com. Natalie, is also from my native home state of Idaho. She is a beautiful person inside and out, and that really comes through in her blogs, programs and videos. Her program with Dr. Monique Middlekauff, "Abs, Core & Pelvic Floor" is what taught me that "less was more" when it came to abdominal exercises and releasing the pelvic floor. Their program really delves into the science as to why.

Unfortunately, just like adenomyosis, diastasis recti is considered as a "non-life-threatening condition." Insurance companies consider it primarily a "cosmetic issue," even though sixty-six percent of patients with a diastasis experience a higher degree of pain in the abdominal and pelvic regions and develop other issues, such as Pelvic Floor Dysfunction, various hernias, muscular-skeletal alignment issues, and even aortic aneurysm. It is because I developed a hernia, that I was able to have the entire procedure covered under insurance. The repair was done laparoscopically in July of 2017, nine days after moving and separating from my husband. After having the surgery, I have noticed a significant difference. I can actually feel my muscles working when I attempt to "suck in my gut." The progress is slow, but again, realizing that my muscles had fifteen years of not being able to work together, it's going to take some practice and some patience. Slow and steady.

Chapter 7:

All We Need

"We don't accomplish anything in this world alone...and whatever happens is the result of the whole tapestry of one's life and all the weavings of individual threads from one to another that creates something."
– Sandra Day O'Connor

The importance of a supportive environment cannot be understated. While society likes to promote a culture of the strength and power of the individual, and that to need help is weak, the truth is that humans are tribal in nature. People automatically struggle when isolated and alone, but when they are encouraged by others they grow faster, and their success amplifies toward others. Even an award-winning athlete doesn't accomplish it alone. He or she has an entire team of coaches and medics, family and fans to support and cheer them on to victory. And nothing is worse than going through chronic pain when you are isolated or alienated by family and/or friends. I was about to face the biggest battle of my life and I felt like I was out on the field alone.

In August of 2014, I lost a dear friend of mine to polycystic ovarian syndrome (PCOS). Less than a year prior, we were having lunch when she told me about her diagnosis and planned treatment. We talked about our "girl problems" for a while and I remember that she told me to never give up on finding answers to my health issues. The morning I learned of her passing; I was devastated. Like me, she was a military spouse with two children. I desperately needed to find answers.

The truth was, I knew deep down that my uterus had to go. It was screaming at me, and it was screaming at me for a long time, I just didn't understand why nobody else could hear it. I had dreams of taking a knife and cutting my uterus out myself in the shower. At the same time, losing an organ and one so central to the female identity, was not an easy decision. I was left questioning what wrong-doing I did to cause my body to turn on me in this way.

In January of 2015, the government insurance policy changed again, and I had an appointment with an OB-GYN recommended by my friend, Heidi. The first meeting was a consult and I handed her my file, about as thick as a dictionary, and told her that I put what I felt were the most relevant notes on top. The doctor smiled and said that she would look it over but would be running her own tests. Yup, I'd heard that before—more poking with needles, more transvaginal ultrasounds, and more invasive pelvic exams. Yippee! Just thinking about the tests got me emotional. I looked at her and pleaded with her, saying, "I know. Just promise me you'll figure out what's wrong because I'm tired of the pain and all the bleeding."

She smiled again and said, "We will figure it out. See you next week."

That following week, I had the lovely pelvic exam and my doctor ordered the ultrasound through the hospital. When the results came back from the ultrasound, they showed an enlarged uterus and a fibroid tumor. My doctor assured me that most fibroids are benign, but we would want to do a biopsy to make sure. She performed a biopsy and gave me a rundown of my options for treatment.

She said I could do nothing and wait for menopause, when most of my issues would just fade away. My second option was to have a uterine ablation, where doctors insert a balloon-like object inside the body and fill it up with heated fluids, searing the fibroid and endometrial tissue off. This procedure usually helps for a while and was basically a band-aid until menopause.

Alternatively, I could have a uterine artery embolization, which cuts off the blood supply to the fibroid and keeps it from growing. As a result, the fibroid will eventually shrink, but that wouldn't address my other problems.

Finally, my doctor mentioned that I could have a hysterectomy and just take the whole thing out. I told her I was leaning towards the complete removal option but wanted to talk to my husband about it first. She said, "No rush. We'll talk about it more when we get your biopsy results back."

Then, handing me back my file, she said, "I almost hate to tell you this, but I looked at this, and this ultrasound done back in 2008 shows that your uterus was enlarged back then. It seems they didn't know what they were looking at because they said it was 'unremarkable,' but that's about the size of a pregnant woman at three-four months gestation."

I felt anger and rage well up inside me as she told me this. Did she say that I could have been spared seven years of pain if these people knew what they were looking at?

When Guy got home that evening, I shared all this information with him, telling him I finally had a diagnosis, what my options were, and that I was leaning towards the hysterectomy and my reasoning for this, but

I wanted to know his thoughts. Guy didn't have a lot of input, even about what the doctor said about the ultrasound done by the military back in 2008. It was as if he didn't care and it was my problem to figure out alone.

In April 2015, I went back to get my biopsy results and she said they were "inconclusive." I sat there and asked, "What does that mean?" My doctor explained that the tissue that was tested had some abnormal cells, but that didn't mean that it was cancer, but she couldn't rule it out either. She could do another biopsy, but she really didn't want to put me through that again, especially since I was electing to do a hysterectomy. "We can just biopsy it then, once it's out," she informed me, and ordered an MRI, just to get another perspective on everything and told me to let her know when I was ready to schedule my surgery.

The plan was to do the hysterectomy laparoscopically, so that there would be a quicker heal time than with my c-sections. But if there were any complications, I would need to be opened up, so I had to be prepared for the more invasive procedure, which meant a four-week minimum recovery with a possible six to eight weeks.

When Guy got home, I told him about the biopsy. Naturally, I was freaking out because I read about inconclusive biopsies online and he said, "Inconclusive just means they don't know. What do you think it means?"

I said, "I think it means fifty-fifty chance. I'm not going to know until it's out anyway."

"So, I wouldn't worry about it," Guy said.

Not worrying was probably a healthy way of looking at it because worrying would not change anything, but I felt like Guy was minimizing my concerns. My father died of abdominal cancer, and he had a "jelly belly" that stuck out like a pregnant woman. I was freaking out.

When I asked Guy if there was a time that worked best for him to schedule my surgery, so he could get time off to help with the kids, he said he didn't think he could get time off.

"Ugh," I thought, "here we go again. Third time is a charm. I'm going to have a surgery, there will be complications, I'll have to spend a week in the hospital and he's not going to be around to help during recovery."

First thing I did was call Guy's mom to see if she would be available to come out sometime that summer. Unfortunately, she didn't know because they had their dogs and were moving her mom and had lots of things going on. She suggested maybe I could have the surgery out there in Idaho because military people did it all the time. I appreciated her ideas and then went down my list.

Both of my sisters had busy work schedules, and certainly couldn't cover my recovery time if it lasted six to eight weeks. It was hard to live over 2,000 miles away from your family when major life events like these came up. As I talked to my doctor about the possibility of having the surgery out in Idaho, she said that I couldn't file with insurance to have the procedure done in two different states at the same time, but since I didn't want to have the hysterectomy done until summer, when my kids were out of school, I had some time to investigate the prospect of having the surgery done there.

I found a surgeon in Boise, who accepted our insurance and was available, but I had to make an appointment to see him first, so that he could corroborate that the surgery was necessary. After that, he would have to schedule the hysterectomy with the hospital, which would take two to four weeks from our first appointment. I soon realized that if I ended up requiring a full abdominal hysterectomy, I would not be recovered in time to have the kids back in Virginia for the upcoming school year.

"Ugh," I thought, "This isn't going to work. What am I going to do? I'll just schedule the surgery here and hope someone can come out and help, and if they can't then I'll just have to pray that everything goes well, and I can handle things on my own.

Guy became increasingly frustrated and angry with me, accusing me of putting off my surgery by pursuing the idea of having it in Idaho, which was his mother's suggestion initially. So I did not understand why he was so mad at me. Aside from that, Guy didn't seem to appreciate that I was trying to make sure the needs of our children were being met, if anything went wrong during my surgery. It wasn't like I had a great track record with abdominal surgeries, so I just wanted all the bases covered. Lastly, it still concerned me that Guy minimized my fears of having a biopsy that was "inconclusive." It frightened me that my surgery was going to require the assistance of an oncologist. This fact also made scheduling the surgery a bit more complicated because it required working around an additional doctor's schedule.

On July 14, 2015, I found Guy's wedding ring left on his bedside table. When he got home from work that day, I placed it back on his finger, assuming he forgot to put it on after doing yoga or something. The next day, I noticed his bedside table drawer slightly open, and saw his ring inside the drawer. This was not accidental. When I confronted Guy about it, his explanation for not wearing his wedding band was, "It didn't feel right." Hearing those words was like a knife to my heart. I was going to be going into surgery in a matter of weeks, and I didn't know whether my husband was going to be by my side or not. I was hysterical. I remember asking him if there was someone else, and he denied that there was. I remember saying that I was sorry for getting injured giving birth to our children, but I needed him to be my rock through this surgery and I demanded that he put his ring back on. He refused.

Right around this same time I received a phone call from Guy's cousin, Rachel, in New York City, who wanted to check on me. She and I had shared some "girl problem" conversations during our annual Thanksgiving visits. But this time she was calling because it had come through the family grapevine to her that I was "unbearable to be around." Being that she and I got along like sisters, she knew that didn't sound like me and wanted to reach out. The fact that I was the subject of some negative coastal rumor mill was frustrating. There was only one place this story could have originated from and that was my husband. Whether he confided in his mom, or his sister, or whoever, it was now sweeping the Pacific Northwest and made its way to the East Coast. I decided to put an end to the rumors and air out my entire "I may or may not have cancer and I'm having my womb removed in a week" on Facebook for all my friends to read. Most of the family responded by saying "I had no idea," and wished me well. I had several friends confide that they had been through something similar in the past and lent me their words of support and encouragement.

August 4, 2015 arrived—the day of my surgery. Besides the fibroid tumor and the adenomyosis of the uterus, I also had severe pelvic adhesive disease, resulting in my bladder becoming attached to my uterus, as well as my left ovary, small bowel, and other organs all attached to my left abdominal wall. If you recall, that Velcro-like tearing I experienced the year prior, that was on my left side, so yes, my adhesions were real. My bladder was injured during the surgery and my doctor feared she would have to do a full abdominal incision to repair it and to remove the other adhesions. Luckily, she allowed the oncologist, who was also a skilled laparoscopic surgeon, to try to repair this before she opened me up. The oncologist was able to complete my surgery laparoscopically. I ended up staying the night in the hospital, as the surgery went longer than originally intended. I went home the next day still with a catheter in. The main thing I remember was waking up from the anesthesia and no longer feeling that "bowling ball" in my stomach. I knew immediately that having the hysterectomy was the right decision. When my doctor came by to check on me, I remember her saying, "You were a real mess in there. I don't know how you were functioning." This was the validation I needed. All the pain I had felt was real. I wasn't crazy and I didn't make it up.

I had follow-up appointments the next two days, for which I was grateful that my mother-in-law was able to make it out. She drove me to my appointments because Guy had to work. Even though he wasn't at my follow-up appointments, where my doctors instructed me to start weaning off the opioids, Guy made it a point when he was home from work to dictate to me about how and when I was to take my pain medication. I don't remember exactly what I said in front of his mother, because I was on drugs, but it was probably to the tune of "You weren't at my appointment, so how would you know. Go shut up and don't tell me what to do." I was angry, because he still refused to wear his wedding band, and I'm pretty sure he didn't even try to get the time off from work. Work was an excuse. I really thought that having all my pain proven by these doctors that Guy's fears would be pacified, and he could find the compassion to understand what I had been feeling and forgive me for whatever story he was telling himself. But no, it appeared he was still upset with me about something.

This was particularly difficult because I wasn't in the most encouraging environment for healing. My husband would accuse me of "lashing out" occasionally, and I admittedly would "lash out" if I was scared and was being "encouraged" or manipulated into doing something he wanted me to do that I believed was going to cause me pain. And as experience would dictate, after giving in to his encouragement on multiple occasions in the past, it usually did cause me great pain.

He also had his episodes of rage, what his sister referred to as "channeling Fred," referring to their father. I never met their father. He died about six months after I had moved back to Boise from working with Southwest Airlines in Phoenix, Arizona. But I can only assume that their dad exhibited explosive tantrums, and this was a tolerated behavior, that I unfortunately was all too familiar with, as my dad occasionally did the same thing if we kids didn't do what was expected. It was as if I was living back under my father's roof again, getting yelled at because dinner wasn't on the table, the house was a mess with his "to do piles," or the laundry didn't get done and it's my fault that I'm still in chronic pain, or that I parked the car ten inches too close to the basketball pole that forced him to ram his car into the side of mine. Yes, that was one of my favorite episodes (sarcasm.) I feel that I did my best to tolerate these tantrums because I knew he was under a lot of stress at work, and that his anger really wasn't about me, even though he liked to project it onto me.

After the first week of recovery was under my belt, his mother flew back to Idaho with the kids for a two-week visit. Granted, I didn't have to look after the kids and I could rest, but I also didn't have any helping hands around, who could grab things from upstairs for me, if I wanted or needed assistance. I was home all alone, one week after a pretty traumatic surgery.

Luckily, I felt so much better with my uterus gone that I recovered relatively quickly and started to get my energy back. By my six-week follow-up, my doctor said I was healing well and was able to return to "normal activity." Guy and I had sex for the first time in over a year. It was an emotional experience for me because it was almost like being a virgin again, and it was such a relief that it didn't hurt, and I didn't cramp or bleed afterward. For the first time in almost a decade, I had hope that I could be a whole person again and that things would be better with Guy. I believed that Guy shared that hope too, because on several occasions after he left me notes, for example: "I love you, period. Unconditionally, unquestioning, unwavering, forever. Love, your Guy (P.S. thank you for understanding. Dinner was quick, light, and perfect. Only wish it was with you. I'm headed upstairs hoping you are awake)."

Just prior to our fifteenth wedding anniversary, on September 30, Guy proposed we put our wedding bands back on. I was so happy that we were going to have a fresh start. Sadly, this feeling wouldn't last. All of the physical and emotional stress of the past year did not serve me well. As I would later discover, I had stored it in my body, and it manifested into anxiety and anger.

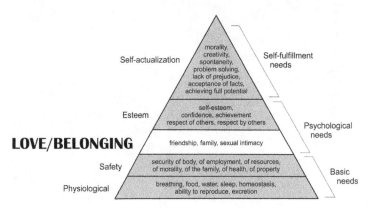

Chapter 8:

Lay Me Down to Sleep

"Any idiot can face a crisis—it's day to day living that wears you out."
– Anton Chekhov

When you suffer from chronic pain, it is difficult to get comfortable enough to sleep as it is. I experienced shocks that would run down my legs at night when I tried to relax, and I had to sleep with my head propped up on a large incline because my enlarged uterus would put pressure on my diaphragm, affecting my breathing. In an attempt to get a restful sleep, which sadly didn't normally happen, I would often take pain meds at night. One night, I was so tired, and after being awoken by my husband, I wrote this poem. Writing has always been an outlet for me to express my thoughts and emotions, and I know those of you suffering from restless sleep and chronic pain can share in this hardship.

I desire a place where I can safely sleep,
Where idling hands cannot wake and creep.
After a long, exhausting day, dormancy is bliss,
Not a caress or a fondle, a stroke or a kiss.
I desire a place where I can safely slumber,
Where roaming hands cannot encroach or encumber.
After a long, tiring day, sleep is my body's only desire,
Not a straying hand, slipping beneath my nightly attire.
I desire a place where I can safely rest,
Where meandering hands cannot touch my breast.
After a long, weary day, my mind and body
need to recover,
Mr. Sandman is my only bedtime lover.

When it comes to sleep, consistency is key. Making sleep a priority is essential. When we sleep, we heal—physically, emotionally and spiritually. If we don't get the right amount of sleep, we are tired, in pain, cranky, and studies show that we are slower, dumber, and even live shorter lives when chronically sleep-deprived.

The one thing I craved more than anything, when suffering from chronic pain, was sleep. I wanted to crawl in bed and sleep for a week, a month, or an even longer stretch of time. I felt burned out and exhausted. When your body is attempting to fight infections, heal injuries, or maintain a level of activity on low reserves, it needs time to recharge, just like a cell phone. If we don't "plug in" for a few hours, occasionally, we are going to run out of bars.

The average person needs six to eight hours of sleep per night. Just like there are saliva tests to find out what foods you should eat, you can also find out how much sleep you need, and this test is scientifically based on your genes. Not everyone is created equal, our genes are programmed with a circadian rhythm, which is why "early birds" and "night owls" both exist. Historically, people would take a daily siesta in the afternoon, around two or three p.m. I know I usually hit a lull around four p.m. every day when working. Our instinct is to grab a snack or cup of coffee to make it through the day—this is a bad idea. Instead, try to take a fifteen-minute walk in the sunshine or a twenty-minute power nap if you can. Drinking caffeine after two or three p.m. will affect your late-night sleep, as does exercising at night, or electronics/screens that give off blue light. Other obstacles to a good night's sleep include sharing your bed with another person or a pet.

Following my hernia surgery in 2017, my surgeon had asked if I was ever diagnosed with sleep apnea or been part of a sleep study. Guy mentioned before that I snored sometimes, but I associated it with my seasonal allergies and never considered my abdominal issues were affecting my sleep also. But when you think about when a woman is pregnant, how that big belly affects everything, from your breathing to your bladder, it makes sense. And it all has to do with the pressure on your pelvic floor muscles. The diaphragm and your pelvic floor muscles have a symbiotic relationship. When you breathe in and your diaphragm elevates, so does your pelvis. When you breathe out, your diaphragm descends and so do your pelvic floor muscles.

Some things that really helped with my sleep, were first getting a fitness band that measures your sleep patterns. I use a Fitbit that tracks not only steps, but my heart rate and sleep as well. It has been so insightful. You will know that you are on the right track with your health when you see your sleep patterns normalize and you feel better in the mornings.

Using meditations before sleep under the direction of your physician, can help regulate your breathing and clear your mind for peaceful dreams and quality sleep. Create an environment that is conducive to sleeping. Use your senses to discern what you need. How does your mattress feel? Perhaps use a weighted blanket. The temperature of the room? What do you hear? If you live near railroad tracks, maybe use a sound machine. What do you see? On full moons, the light can keep one awake. Try using blackout curtains or an eye mask. What do you smell? Spritzing a little lavender on your pillow can set the tone for a calming night.

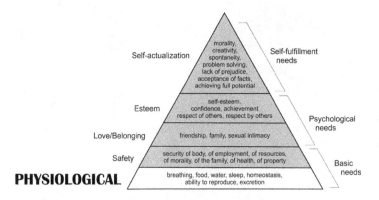

Chapter 9:

Environmental Factors

"It is curious that physical courage
should be so common in the world
and moral courage so rare."
— Mark Twain, *Eruption: Hitherto Unpublished Pages*
About Men and Event (1940)

had mentioned in an earlier chapter that I had started seeing a chiropractor in 2008, when it seemed that my issues were not OB-GYN related. I gave a set of the x-rays to a local chiropractor and he said that my pelvis appeared tilted /rotated forward. After just a couple of appointments with him adjusting my alignment, my sciatic nerve pain running down my leg was virtually gone.

He also noticed my edema, inflammation, and poor core stability and recommended some simple exercises and encouraged drinking lots of water. He also recommended that I see an allergist to determine what might be causing my inflammation, and said most disease stems from the gut, so the cause could be related to food or my environment. I have continued to see him off and on for the last decade, as he was one of the few doctors, who listened and seemed to genuinely care. How ironic that many insurance companies don't cover chiropractic care. In my experience the chiropractors I saw back home in Boise and out here in Virginia would listen to their patients and naturally tried to relieve the cause of the pain, instead of trying to cover up the symptoms with drugs.

My chiropractor educated me on xenobiotics, which are chemical compounds that are not natural to our body but are often found in our body, and our body cannot process them, so they get stored in our bodies as a toxin. These toxins can disrupt our natural chemical (hormone) balance and throw our body's entire equilibrium out of homeostasis. Considering that my hormones were out of balance, this might explain why my menstrual cycle was out of whack. I decided this was a path worth exploring further.

In this chapter I will cover some of the environmental changes I made and then in the next chapter with regards to the xenobiotics in our food/diet.

Since moving to Virginia over a decade ago, I have suffered from seasonal allergies, as do a lot of people. The

East Coast is notorious for the pollen that makes people feel miserable. Interestingly, after having my hysterectomy in 2015, the following Spring, I did not experience the headaches, sneezing, and watery eyes that I usually did. Meanwhile, others still were and spoke about what a terrible Spring it was for pollen. It was at that time that I truly saw the connection. My body was so busy fighting off the infection in my uterus, that it didn't have the resources to fight off the pollen too. Now that my big uterine problem was gone, my body's immune system no longer struggled to keep the effects of my environment at bay. So, the reverse could also be true. Controlling the offenders in your environment can help to keep your immune system less tasked and your body can maintain its equilibrium.

It is honestly surprising how many things we see, touch, hear and breathe that can elevate a stress response in us.

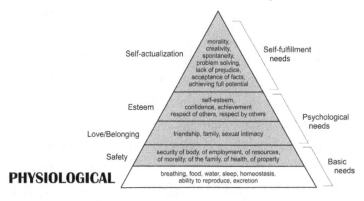

In the air that we breathe, replace the filters on your HVAC system and car regularly.

Wear a mask when using hazardous chemicals like paint or cleaning supplies. Preferably use all-natural, plant-based cleaning products, in your home.

Our skin is our largest organ and we expose it to harmful chemicals all the time, from the detergent we use for washing our clothes and bed sheets, to the soaps, lotions, and cosmetics we apply to our skin daily. Again, being mindful of these products and what is in them and using all-natural body care products will help. Minimizing the use of cosmetics and only using them as socially necessary is honestly the healthiest option.

When it comes to sound pollution, this is one of the things that I really noticed where my body was sensitive. There have been studies on the effects of sound vibrations and the body. It is fascinating really. Loud noises like city traffic and large, noisy crowds can irritate even the healthiest person, but one thing that I noticed that really bothered me was when my husband brushed his teeth. He had a Sonicare toothbrush. There was something about the pitch and sound of it when it vibrated against his teeth that gave me instant headaches. Once I had the hysterectomy the sound didn't give me headaches anymore. For me, this is evidence that if your balance and harmony are already off, your body may be less tolerant of some sounds than a healthier person. This seems to support why people, who are in physical pain, are less patient around loud noises or negative activity.

One of the biggest environmental factors chronic pain patients suffer from is the use of all the pharmaceutical medications. I chose not to take the pain medications I was prescribed on a regular basis, because they would leave me completely non-functional during the day. I only used them at night to help me sleep, especially when the pain level was such that it made it impossible to sleep without them.

I have friends, however, that have had to detox off some of these pain medications, and it is brutal to say the least. One of my friends, Carmen, who has also had multiple surgeries and suffers from both adenomyosis and endometriosis shared her story with me. "I think and hope most of my pain will be resolved when I finally get off these meds. They were helpful and necessary for quite a while, but about two to three years ago, I started noticing that they got less and less effective and more and more detrimental. They sometimes seemed to make my pain worse. I'm pretty sure I have narcotic bowel syndrome and probably opiate-induced hyperalgesia. I started seeing a new pain management specialist in March of 2018. He has helped me tremendously with new cutting-edge treatments that have helped me heal and supported me during this horrendous weaning process. I'm on a restricted diet and using Cannabidiol (CBD), acupuncture, my spinal cord stimulator and various other treatments to help with pain. At the time, I was on a seventy-five mcg/hour fentanyl patch and 120 mg of oxycodone per day. Now I've been off the fentanyl since May 2018 and I'm down to just ten to fifteen mg of oxycodone per day. Every time I've cut my dose it's been awful, especially since one of my withdrawal symptoms is abdominal pain. But eventually my body always adjusts to the lower dose and so I've just kept going drop by drop. It's been hell."

According to the CDC's Division of Reproductive Health, over the last thirty years there has been an accelerated hormone decline in women. From the ages of twenty to forty years, hormone levels plummet thirty to fifty percent. Hormones naturally decline with age, but not at this rate. Research is showing that this acceleration is being caused by our exposure of toxic substances in the environment, these xenobiotics are disrupting our hormones. This may also explain why there is an increase in endometriosis and adenomyosis in women, since both diseases are estrogen driven.

Through learning about energy medicine, I embraced the notion that we are vibrational energy, not just our physical body, and we can concentrate our strength to weak areas of our bodies. Everything in nature gives off a biofield. Energy medicine teaches because our bodies carry so many environmental toxins that are essentially "free radicals" that if we take a break and walk in nature, barefoot in the grass, or hug a tree, it will work like a magnet and help neutralize our biofield. I know that I feel better when I walk in the mountains surrounded by trees. Luckily, I have a preserved park right up the road from me where I can walk. Keeping plants in your home and/or having pets can also help.

Chapter 10:

Diet...It's Not a Fad; It's a Lifestyle.

"High-tech tomatoes. Mysterious milk. Super squash. Are we supposed to eat this stuff? Or is it going to eat us?"
– Anita Manning

T hanks to my chiropractor, who practices whole-body health, I was awakened to the fact that my food consumption and environment could be causing the inflammation in my body. He had recommended that I see a food allergist, however she was booked up solid, so he offered to help me with my personal "investigation." I would like to reiterate that I

91

share my personal story for educational and informational purposes only and in no way should it be considered as or replace qualified medical advice, diagnosis or treatment. It is imperative that any type of diet, particularly of this magnitude be under the supervision of a medical practitioner.

When suffering from pelvic inflammation, one side effect is loss of appetite. When one is in pain, one can feel nauseous or occasionally vomit. In the case of chronic pelvic pain, when one suffers over a long period, you can become malnourished or nutritionally hungry. The body will store fat as a survival trigger, which activates cortisol and affects your metabolism, and there begins the vicious cycle of hardly eating and putting on weight, and not being able to lose the weight. No matter how healthy you think you're eating or how few calories you may be consuming, you cannot lose weight. Your metabolism just shuts down. And if you are like me, and your hormones are out of balance, you can develop hypothyroidism or Hashimoto's Thyroiditis. This can be diagnosed by testing the antibodies in your blood. It is because of this diagnosis, that I have primarily been following the Hashimoto's Protocol for diet.

A suppressed appetite isn't necessarily a bad thing, but rather something to be conscious of, and carefully consider the time of day you eat and how much you consume. Eating at the same time and developing a rhythm is beneficial. Changing up what and how much you eat can keep your metabolism hopping. This kind of mindful awareness helps you to eat smart. I found that the key to eating when you don't "feel hungry" is to eat anyway— just eat small and eat often. Eat something every two to four hours, even if it is just a few carrot sticks or a handful of berries, because this keeps your system active, because mine was "sluggish."

There are all kinds of theories on "diet," and before you try any diet you should consult your doctor and see what resonates with you and your specific situation. To begin, my chiropractor recommended a food elimination diet and detox to see what food sensitivities I had. I admit, the elimination diet wasn't easy, and it wasn't fun, but I learned a lot about myself. The worst part is that during the initial three-day detox, you don't eat anything. You can drink water, herbal teas with no sugar, and take nutritional supplements. During this time, I experienced headaches from lack of caffeine and/or sugar, but after those three days, the headaches faded. On day four, I introduced some fresh and organic/ locally grown greens and see how my body reacted to them. After a couple of days, I introduced some berries or an apple, depending on the season. Again, fresh and organic/locally grown is best. After another few days, I indulged in a protein like local fresh eggs. Then some chicken breast meat or white fish. This process helps you determine how your body reacts to certain foods. Introducing one food at time for a couple of days and listening to your body's reaction to it is the most direct and accurate way to determine what foods are right for you. It is an extensive and arduous process though. I discovered that my body did not like corn, several dairy products, and pork.

Another one of my doctors informed me how heritage can affect food selection. For example, my ancestors were primarily from the Baltic region and were fishermen. It just so happens that I do love fish, especially salmon, and yes, I eat it regularly, but am mindful of it being fresh-caught and where. By taking a DNA test that includes health and diet information, you can find out your DNA cell's genetic predisposition. Eating according to what your ancestors ate makes perfect sense to me and explains why I was sensitive to things like pork, corn and certain cheeses.

Another theory on proper diet is eating seasonally. Our ancestors didn't always have access to certain foods during certain times of the year. For example, eating squash (an autumn harvest food) naturally signals your body that "winter is coming" and you need to store food. This concept is central to Ayurvedic Medicine, one of the world's oldest holistic healing practices. It centers around the five basic elements of the universe, space, air, fire, water and earth. These elements then combine in the human body to form three primary energies or "doshas" with two different dominant element combinations that drive your body's energy. These doshas are Vata (air and space), Pitta (fire and water) and Kapha (water and earth.)

I had taken dosha quizzes online and on paper in the past and usually came out fairly even, to the point I might be what is referred to as "Tridoshic." When I read the qualities of each dosha, I identified primarily with the Vata and Pitta doshas. During this past year, I had the opportunity to meet with a certified ayurvedic practitioner, whom conducted a pulse assessment referred to as Nadi Pariksha. Your pulse diagnosis allows the practitioner to determine your doshic constitution and can then recommend diet and lifestyle practices to restore balance. She determined that I was dual-doshic, both Vata and Pitta, as I had suspected. And most of her dietary recommendation coincided with those of my detox diet and my DNA.

The use of herbs in cooking has had medicinal benefits for centuries. However, most of the herbs we use for cooking are dried, which loses much of the healing quality. The health benefits are in the oils. Therefore, I started cooking with essential oils. Using essential oils in your cooking and baking is amazing because although you lose some of the potency when the oils are subjected to heat, you still enjoy the boost of flavor. One receives the greatest benefits in using them in smoothies and salad dressings, when the oils are not cooked. Or if you add the oil just prior to serving, like adding basil in a tomato sauce, then it is perfect. I love the website www.allthenourishingthings.com hosted by the amazing Lindsey Dietz. She shares fantastic recipes and tips on using the right amount, as it usually only takes a drop, because essential oils are incredibly potent. It is also important to note that not all essential oils are for internal consumption, like wintergreen, so please do your research before cooking with any essential oils. I have included a list of essential oils used in aromatherapy in the resource section at the back of the book for your convenience.

When it comes to losing weight, experts say that ninety-five percent depends on what we consume and only five percent is related to exercise. Basically, our food is our fuel, and this begs the question, do we really know what we are putting into our bodies? Here are some general tips.

Read the labels on your food, and if you can't pronounce an ingredient, don't eat it.

Avoid natural or artificial flavors or colors and watch your sugar intake.

Eat fresh and organic/locally grown whole foods whenever possible.

Chapter 11:

The Beginning of the End

"Do not fight against pain; do not fight against irritation or jealousy. Embrace them with great tenderness as though you were embracing a little baby. Your anger is yourself, and you should not be violent toward it. The same thing goes for all your emotions."
– Thich Nhat Hanh

Reflecting on the quote from Thich Nhat Hanh above, I realized rejecting my feelings ironically fueled my depression, because suffering is just suppressed pain. Meditation and mindfulness techniques allow one to be more aware of their environment and can sometimes produce opposite effects on a trauma survivor. Trauma survivors don't need more awareness, they need to feel safe and secure in their environment. I came to realize that I still didn't feel safe in my body and at times, I didn't even feel safe around my husband.

Although a year passed since my hysterectomy and I was doing physical therapy two or three times a week religiously, I still felt like something wasn't quite right in my body. And that was because I also had the undiagnosed diastasis of the abdominal muscles. Anytime I felt a muscle cramp, particularly in my abdomen, I panicked.

I began going to yoga classes again in May 2016 and would occasionally have feelings of panic/anxiety. The instructor had experience with clients suffering from PTSD and recognized it in me. Nearly ten percent of women with a pregnancy complication meet the full criteria for PTSD and approximately thirty percent meet partial criteria. Though some women recover within a year, about one-third of women develop chronic symptoms. Most people associate PTSD with soldiers or wounded warriors, but you don't have to be injured on a battlefield to be a wounded warrior. You could be injured in a hospital bed bringing a baby into the world. Anxiety can be triggered by any internal or external stressor, because it is your body's stress response system reacting to a perceived threat in the present or future but learned from the past.

In March of 2016, I completed an online course on "Mindfulness for Wellbeing and Peak Performance" through Monash University. Mindfulness, is the scientific concept of being aware of your surroundings. For example, there is a ladder and an item on the top shelf that you need and in order to obtain it you need to be present in that moment. You are going to climb that ladder and get it, not be stuck in the past telling yourself that because you had a c-section you are broken and you can't climb that ladder; or anticipate the fear of the future and tell yourself that if you step up that ladder you are going to lose your balance and fall and break a bone. It's recognizing your thoughts and feelings and not dismissing your fears but acknowledging them, thanking them for wanting to protect you and saying, "we will be all right," and taking the steps needed to feel safe and climb that ladder and get what you need.

There are dozens of meditation apps that are available to download on your phone. Most offer a free limited trial and then a full use subscription. I encourage you to try a few of them out first to see what style is best for you. Two of my favorites are Headspace and Ten Percent Happier, because they include meditations for mornings and some specifically for before bedtime. Starting out your day with a quick five to ten-minute meditation, especially after waking up to a startling alarm clock (if you are like many and that is how you normally wake up,) will calm your system and allow you to focus on your day in a more productive fashion. It is so much healthier than the rushed scramble that tends to be today's normal.

Another practice I was introduced to for anxiety was Emotional Freedom Technique (EFT) or "Tapping." Tapping is essentially a form of self-reflexology, using pressure points.

I will be honest, in that at first, I thought it was a bit silly and simple, but it really does help calm me. Like the meditation apps available on your phone, there are several "Tapping" ones also. I use the "Tapping Solutions" app.

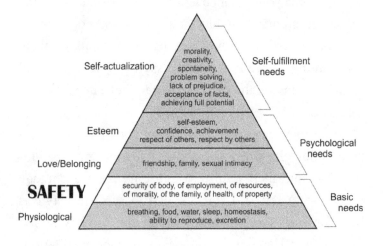

Chapter 12:

One Last Gift

*"Be more concerned with your character
than with your reputation. Your character
is what you are while your reputation is
merely what others think you are."*
– Dale Carnegie, *How to Win Friends &
Influence People (1936)*

April 5, 2017, marked over six months since
my last appointment with my surgeon, and I
didn't see any more progress in doing physical therapy with regards to my stomach muscles. My
doctor acknowledged that my abdominal muscles were
still weak and noticed a bit of a gap between them,

giving me a referral to a specialist. Upon seeing the specialist, I learned that I developed a hernia and would require another surgery to repair it and the gap between my abdominal muscles. I called Guy at work, extremely emotional. While I was glad that I had an explanation as to why the exercises weren't helping, I was not at all happy about the idea of having another abdominal surgery. Guy assured me that everything would be fine, and that we would get through it. I felt better after talking to him.

That evening, the home phone rang, and it was CVS Pharmacy. I was in the pharmacy earlier that day, so I answered the phone assuming it was for me. But the person on the phone asked for Guy.

After saying, "This is Guy," he then walked out of the front door, and in a raised voice, I heard him say, "Why are you calling me on this number?" After a few minutes, he walked back inside. It wasn't uncommon for Guy to walk outside to take a phone call because cell phone reception was often better outdoors, but this call was on the landline, and this call was from a pharmacist. Guy was never sick. I was concerned and asked him if he was okay, to which he replied, "Yes," and said they just called to verify insurance information.

For the remainder of the evening, Guy did not seem himself. He said he was just tired and wanted to get some rest, which was not like him either. I was worried but didn't press any further.

The next morning, on Thursday, April 6, 2017, Guy called me while he was at work and told me that he was having an affair, and that he tested positive for chlamydia, and that I needed to get myself checked. I didn't get angry and yell at him. I remember saying that I appreciated him telling me because I was sure it was a difficult thing for him to confess. Guy responded, saying, "You do love me," as if he doubted that I did. I said we could talk about this when he got home, but I wanted to call my doctor straight away and see if I could get an appointment. I was able to get an appointment that afternoon and had myself tested for everything. Words cannot describe the humiliation of being tested for a sexually transmitted disease, when you thought you were in a committed relationship. I was truly mortified. The nurse told me it would take about a week for the results to come back, which meant that his "girlfriend" warned him about a week prior. My doctor immediately prescribed me an antibiotic, since it was likely that I also contracted the disease because we were sexually active over the last month.

That evening, we spoke only briefly about the affair. I asked him who it was with, and he said it wasn't important. I told him that it was important to me, particularly if it was with someone who I knew. I asked him if it was an employee; he said it wasn't. I asked him if it was someone from the yoga studio, or his fraternity; he said that it wasn't. Instead, he told me that it was someone that he met online. At first, I felt relief at that notion, but the more I thought about it, I came to realize that it meant his affair wasn't a chance meeting, but was rather a planned, intentional meeting. That was heartbreaking.

We were scheduled to fly home to Boise together as a family, for spring break (April 14 to 22), but the trip ended up just being with me and the kids. I stayed in Guy's mother's house not saying a word about his infidelity while taking medication for the subsequent yeast infection that developed from the antibiotics I had to take because of his indiscretion. I had a follow up with my doctor upon my return on April 24 and found out that I tested positive for a bacterial infection and would need to be retested in about three months to make sure that the antibiotics worked.

Guy minimized my pain again because he was healthy, he didn't experience any symptoms, he took the antibiotic, and he was all good. He didn't understand how a curable STI like Chlamydia could be a problem for me. First of all, there is the issue that I have an autoimmune disease. There is a reason I developed an autoimmune disease, because my body has been fighting off infections constantly for years. I have been subjected to so many antibiotics it's just not even funny. All the surgeries, the breast infections, ear infections, UTI's with my damaged bladder, yeast infections, the list just goes on and on and on. Second, I had a hysterectomy. I no longer have my cervix protecting the entrance of my vagina. Yup, my front door was just wide open. STI's cause inflammation of the sensitive mucosa of the vagina. When this tissue is compromised due to an infection, it's easier for another microorganism to enter the body and begin to grow. This is why all of my recurring episodes are categorized as Bacterial Vaginosis (BV), which is essentially an overgrowth of bad bacteria that throws off the natural balance of the vagina. As usual, the cause and cure of BV is not entirely understood but certain activities like unprotected sex increase your risk. Unlike some infections, in which a person develops immunity after exposure, the body does not develop any immunity against chlamydia after an infection. Chlamydia can lie dormant in the body for many years, causing a low-grade infection without symptoms. It could potentially flare up causing a symptomatic infection, especially if there was an alteration in my immune system, such as a severe cold, flu, cancer, or some other severe illness. After texting Guy the link to a scientific article about how Chlamydia can hide in your gastrointestinal tract, after I've taken antibiotics three times for this crap, his response was "Interesting." That's it.

Clearly, there was no remorse expressed there in his text, how his actions have affected me. He knew about my fragile health situation, he cheated, and his failure to use condoms demonstrated a lack of care. The more I tried to explain how this was affecting me the more he blew me off. If you talk too much about your illness and how it affects you, people may think you're being negative or letting your illness define you, but if you don't talk about your illness, people won't understand what you are going through. This can often seem like a double-edged sword, and it is important to differentiate between talking about your illness and complaining about it. However, even if a person is complaining about their illness, they still deserve to be witnessed and receive compassion.

The damages from an STD can be life-altering, including lifelong medical expenses and an increased risk of cancer. Chlamydia has been linked to Pelvic Inflammatory Disease, which can then lead to a host of problems. My doctors are still monitoring lesions that have developed on my left side near my spleen. Such a lovely parting gift.

Many individuals who contract an STD experience emotional distress such as depression, guilt and isolation. I'm all too familiar with those symptoms, dealing with the grief of having a hysterectomy. When talking to my parish priest, he said that because he knew the faithful and loyal person I am, he knew that I would never give up on Guy. The only way I could be free from our unbalanced marriage was for him to betray me. Strangely, that made sense to me.

The philosopher Immanuel Kant said that lying was always morally wrong. Dignity is based on the concept that humans are capable of freely making their own decisions and guiding their conduct by reason, to be ethical and respect the power in oneself and others. Understanding this, lies are morally wrong for two reasons. For one, lies corrupt the important quality of being human, and your ability to make free choices. Each lie contradicts the part of you that gives you moral worth. Secondly, lies rob others of their freedom to choose. Telling a lie leads people to decide differently than they would have had they known the truth. It's a way of controlling or manipulating an outcome. I came to realize that Guy had a lot of secrets and lies, not just as a spouse but as his business partner and co-parent. Forgiveness will not come easy.

This is another poem I composed, as I sat and identified all the feelings I needed to release.

FEEL
Pain, loss, grief
Disease, surgery, relief
Trauma, anger, repression
Fear, anxiety, depression
Betrayal, isolation, shame
Excuses, lies, blame
My sacred space infected
By his insecurities projected
These emotions are valid and real
In honoring each one I heal

Healing. That is what this book is all about. For me it has been healing to get my thoughts and feelings out of my head and on to paper. Sharing my story is easier believing that it brings some sort of purpose to the suffering; that sharing what I have learned could prevent others from having the same negative experience or let them know that they are not crazy or alone in their struggle. My HOPE is that everyone, who comes across my book will learn that whatever is causing your chronic pain, whether by trauma our autoimmune disease, you can analyze your exercise, sleep, environment and diet, and make adjustments that will improve your life. May we all be healthy, happy and healed.

Aromatherapy Resource

Essential Oil	Healing Properties
Basil	Supports digestion, headache/muscle pain reliever
Bergamot	Disinfectant, reduces stress
Black Pepper	Supports digestion, headache/muscle pain reliever
Cardamom	Antimicrobial, antiseptic
Cassia	Antimicrobial, immunity
Cedarwood	Balances menstrual cycle
Chamomile	Reduces anxiety, inflammation, nausea, indigestion
Cilantro	Supports digestion, heals skin irritations, immunity
Cinnamon	Boosts circulation, relieves congestion
Clary Sage	supports digestion
Clove	Antibacterial, antioxidant, reduces inflammation
Eucalyptus	Improves respiration, purification
Fennel	Supports digestion, muscle pain reliever
Frankincense	Builds immunity, reduces inflammation
Geranium	Aids in urination

Ginger	Relieves nausea, reduces inflammation
Grapefruit	Supports metabolism and cellulite reduction
Helichrysum	Supports digestion
Jasmine	Antiseptic, reduces inflammation
Juniper	Antiseptic, reduces inflammation
Lavender	Promotes relaxation, heals skin irritations
Lemon	Antibacterial, boosts immunity
Lemongrass	Relaxes muscles, calms the mind
Melissa	Antibacterial, emotional balance
Melaleuca	Antibacterial, Antifungal
Myrrh	Antiseptic, reduces inflammation
Orange	Improves libido, anti-inflammatory
Oregano	Antimicrobial, heals scars
Palo Santo	Antibacterial, anti-inflammatory
Peppermint	Supports digestion, headache/muscle pain reliever
Rose	Reduces inflammation
Rosemary	Clarity, improves brain function/memory
Sandalwood	Improves libido, anti-inflammatory

Sweet Marjoram	Improves respiration, muscle pain reliever
Tarragon	Improves circulation
Thyme	Antiseptic, reduces inflammation
Vanilla	Antibacterial
Vetiver	Heals scars
Wintergreen	Antiseptic, muscle pain reliever
Ylang Ylang	Antimicrobial

Recommendations by the Author for Further Exploration

(Spiritual Healing)

Dunn, B. & Leonard, K. (2004). *Through a Season of Grief: Devotions for your journey from mourning to joy.* Nashville, TN: Thomas Nelson Inc.

Estés, C. (2011). *Untie the Strong Woman: Blessed Mother's Immaculate Love for the Wild Soul.* Boulder, CO: Sounds True Inc.

Hoffman, N. (2018). *Is it Me? Making Sense of Your Confusing Marriage: A Christian Woman's Guide to Hidden Emotional and Spiritual Abuse.* Rosemount, MN: Flying Free Media.

Popcak, G. (2011). *The Life God Wants You to Have: Discovering the Divine Plan When Human Plans Fail.* New York, NY: The Crossroad Publishing Company.

Trimm, C. (2014). *PUSH: Persevere Until Success Happens through prayer.* Shippensburg, PA: Destiny Image Publishers Inc.

Worwood, V. (2006). *Aromatherapy for the Soul: Healing the Spirit with Fragrance and Essential Oils.* Novato, CA: New World Library.

(Physical Healing)

Breus, M. (2016). *The Power of When: Discover Your Chronotype and the Best Time to Eat Lunch, Ask for a Raise, Have Sex, Write a Novel, Take Your Meds, and More.* New York, NY: Little, Brown and Company.

Bowman, K. (2016). *Diastasis Recti: The Whole-Body Solution to Abdominal Weakness and Separation.* Sequim, WA: Propriometricspress.com

Eden, D. & Feinstein, D. (2008). *Energy Medicine: Balancing Your Body's Energies for Optimal Health, Joy and Vitality.* New York, NY: Penguin Group

Finlayson, J. (2019). *You Are What Your Grandparents ATE: What You Need to Know About Nutrition, Experience, Epigenetics & the Origins of Chronic Disease.* Toronto, ON: Robert Rose Inc.

Gregg, S. (2008). *The Complete Illustrated Encyclopedia of Magical Plants.* Beverly, MA: Fair Winds Press

Herrera, I. (2017). *Female Pelvic Alchemy: Trade Secrets for Energizing Your Love Life, Enhancing Your Pleasure & Loving Your Body Completely.* New York, NY: Duplex Publishing.

Malone, S. (2016). *INFLAMED: discover the root cause of inflammation and personalize a step-by-step plan to create a healthy, vibrant life.* Mount Juliet, TN: Agustin Publishing.

Myers, A. (2015). *The Autoimmune Solution: Prevent and Reverse the Full Spectrum of Inflammatory Symptoms and Diseases.* New York, NY: Harper Collins Publishers.

Norman, A. (2018). *Ask Me About My Uterus: A Quest to Make Doctors Believe in Women's Pain.* New York, NY: Nation Books.

Romm, A. (2017). *The Adrenal Thyroid Revolution: A Proven 4-Week Program to Rescue Your Metabolism, Hormones, Mind & Mood.* New York, NY: Harper Collins Publishers.

Weil, A. (2018). *Mind Over Meds: Know When Drugs Are Necessary, When Alternatives Are Better—and When to Let Your Body Heal on Its Own.* New York, NY: Little, Brown and Company.

Wentz, I. (2017). *Hashimoto's Protocol: A 90-Day Plan for Reversing Thyroid Symptoms and Getting Your Life Back.* New York, NY: Harper Collins Publishers.

Yeager, M. (2018). *Why Can't Anyone Help Me? The Nightmare of Adenomyosis.* Middletown, DE: Create Space Independent Publishing.

(Emotional Healing)

Amara, H. & Ruiz, M. (2019). *The Art of Showing Up: Bringing Your True Self to All Your Relationships.* Boulder, CO: Sounds True.

Baker, B. (2018). *Built to Break: When God Writes Your Story and All Hell Breaks Loose.* Enumclaw, WA: Redemption Press.

Brown, B. (2012). *Daring Greatly: How the Courage to Be Vulnerable Transforms the Way We Live, Love, Parent and Lead.* New York, NY: Avery Books.

Brown, R., Gerberg, P. & Muskin, P. (2009). *How to Use Herbs, Nutrients & Yoga in Mental Health.* New York, NY: W.W. Norton & Company.

Callander, M. (2014). *After His Affair: Women Rising from the Ashes of Infidelity.* Asheville, NC: Akasha Publications.

James, J. & Friedman, R. (2009). *The Grief Recovery Handbook: The Action Program for Moving Beyond Death, Divorce, and Other Losses, Including Health, Career, and Faith.* New York, NY: Harper Collins Publishers.

Jinpa, T. (2015). *A Fearless Heart: How the Courage to Be Compassionate Can Transform Our Lives.* New York, NY: Avery Books.

Kogan, N. (2018). *Happier Now: How to Stop Chasing Perfection and Embrace Everyday Moments (Even the Difficult Ones).* Boulder, CO: Sounds True.

Maisel, E. (2012). *Rethinking Depression: How to Shed Mental Health Labels and Create Personal Meaning.* Novato, CA: New World Library.

McGonigal, K. (2012). *The Neuroscience of Change: A Compassion-Based Program for Personal Transformation.* Boulder, CO: Sounds True.

Neff, K. (2013). *Self-Compassion Step by Step: The Proven Power of Being Kind to Yourself.* Boulder, CO: Sounds True.

Northrup, C. (2018). *Dodging Energy Vampires: An Empath's Guide to Evading Relationships that Drain You and Restoring Your Health and Power.* Carlsbad, CA: Hay House, Inc.

Sarkis, S. (2018). *Gaslighting: Recognize Manipulative and Emotionally Abusive People—and Break Free.* New York, NY: Hachette Book Group.

Van Der Kolk, B. (2014). *The Body Keeps The Score.* New York, NY: Penguin Books.

References

Online References

Eveleth, R. (2014). "Chlamydia Can Live in Your Gut and Reinfect You After You're Cured." *Smithsonian. com*: Retrieved from URL
https://www.smithsonianmag.com/smart-news/chlamydia-can-live-your-gut-and-reinfect-you-after-youre-cured-180949688/

Fisher, S. (2017). "Womb: Creation Compassion." *Hebrew Word Lessons*: Retrieved from URL
https://hebrewwordlessons.com/2017/11/26/womb-creation-compassion/

Gimpel, J. (2014). "Father's gene linked to baby's birth weight." *Great Ormond Street Hospital for Children NHS Foundation Trust*: Retrieved from URL
https://www.gosh.nhs.uk/news/latest-press-releases/

2014-press-release-archive/father-s-gene-linked-
baby-s-birth-weight

Website References

Abs, Core & Pelvic Floor / Natalie Hodson
https://nataliehodson.com

Adenomyosis Fighters / Maria Yeager
https://adenofighter.com

All the Nourishing Things / Lindsey Dietz
https://allthenourishingthings.com/

Acknowledgments

To the Author Training Academy: Special thanks to Angela Lauria, CEO & Founder of The Author Incubator for believing in me and my message. To my Developmental Editor, Mehrina Asif, and Managing Editor, Cory Hott, thanks for making the process seamless and keeping me on track. Many more thanks to everyone else at TAI, but especially Cheyenne, Ramses, and Chanelle for their emotional support and guidance.

Thank you to David Hancock and the Morgan James Publishing team for helping me bring this book to print.

To my family, I thank you for all the emotional support and accepting me as I am. Special thanks to my sister, Christine, who flew out for a week to care for me and my children during my last surgery in 2017. Your help was invaluable since we had only moved into the house nine days prior to my hernia surgery. Thank you also for always being willing to be my trivia partner at the Vista Lounge. We must reclaim our title again soon! And to my sister, Cindi, for her feedback on drafts of my book and for creating the graphic images of Maslow's Hierarchy of Needs. Your talent and guidance are greatly appreciated.

To my tribes of friends in the U.S. and abroad, online and in person. Each virtual hug and physical hug, word of kindness, encouragement, or validation of my sanity throughout the years gave me hope and kept me going. There are way too many to mention individually. However, I would like to bring special thanks to those that have shared their personal struggles with women's health issues, especially those whom entrusted me to share some of their stories in this book. To Maria, Carmen & Jennifer, my heartfelt gratitude.

To my doctors and therapists, who listened and cared, and never gave up on finding the root causes to all my pain and assisting in my rehabilitation. I am eternally grateful for giving me my life back. Special thanks to Laurie for sharing her insight and encouragement in putting my thoughts and feelings to paper.

To my amazingly talented friend Lori Diane for taking my headshot photo and making me look good. Lord knows that was not an easy task, especially on a rainy morning. Your ability to make it so easy and willingness to support are truly a blessing.

Finally, to my children. Thank you for all your love and your patience. Living with a parent with chronic pain is not easy, especially when that parent is your primary caregiver and chauffeur. I am so proud of both of you and the incredibly thoughtful, creative, and caring individuals you have grown to become. Thank you for supporting me in telling my story and assisting with the design of my book cover. You two are my everything and I love you to the forest moon of Endor and beyond. Forever.

About the Author

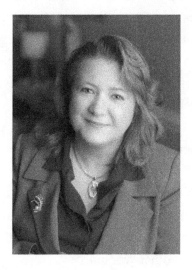

Carolyn Marthanoír is a freelance writer who was first published in her grade school's newspaper. She's been writing ever since.

Carolyn's passion is travel. She graduated with honors from the prestigious Northwest Schools (NWS) of Portland, Oregon, with a focus on airline and travel.

She worked in the travel industry for more than a decade in ground operations and customer service.

Her writing has been published on behalf of various non-profit organizations in the U.S. and U.K. on such topics as military family advocacy and historic preservation. As a U.S. Naval Officer's wife, Carolyn actively applied her writing skills in the promotion of the Military Spouses Residency Relief Act of 2009. Her essay, The Political Battle of the Military Family, received an award in 2010 given by the National Society Daughters of the American Revolution at their 119th Continental Congress in Washington, D.C.

Carolyn's pelvic pain journey began with the pregnancy of her first child, who was born via cesarean section in 2003. Her petite size-six frame ballooned to deliver a child weighing just over eleven pounds. Surviving with multiple "invisible" and undiagnosed conditions for over a decade, she recovered and redirected her energy to help other women.

A recent graduate of Compassion Cultivation Training, developed at the Center for Compassion and Altruism Research and Education (CCARE) at Stanford University, Carolyn assists her clients in developing and executing individualized wellness plans through her one-on-one programs.

Carolyn is a native of Boise, Idaho.